THE
NATURAL CARNIVORE

High Protein Carnivore Diet Cookbook:
the Nutrition for Best Athletic Performance,
Weight Loss and Muscle Growth

Melany Loss Zone

TABLE OF CONTENTS

Introduction

This is the right book for you if you're someone who likes a juicy steak or just about any type of meat. Here we will delve deeply into a diet that questions what you know about nutrition and health and encourages you to explore new possibilities. This diet is the Carnivore Diet, as the title suggests. Many of you may or may not be familiar with the concept of this diet, but it will all be clarified in this book.

The Carnivore Diet's main emphasis is on eating only meat from any source and stopping eating plant food. This diet has recently gained a lot of popularity, and this diet's strong motivation is usually weight loss. Many people follow this diet to resolve a certain form of autoimmune response.

After attempting the Paleo and the Ketogenic diet, many people try the Carnivore diet. The Paleo diet, as you might learn, is a caveman lifestyle that focuses on eating fresh foods like our caveman ancestors ate. It eliminates all processed foods, grains, milk, sugars, etc. that were not available at the time.

When you read the book, you'll grasp the precise ramifications of the carnivore diet. The meat diet alone is very self-explanatory, but there are a few gray areas to building an acceptable healthy diet for yourself. A lot of people have tried this diet, and if properly followed, you will profit from losing weight and becoming healthy. This diet is like a dream come true for you if you're a meat lover.

The Carnivore Diet is a special type of diet consisting of animal produced foods which exempts vegetables and legumes. Also, you can eat things like yogurt, cheese, and milk alongside the Carnivore Diet. For some people, they do not like the Carnivore Diet because it is not good for their respective health. However, to other people, they have been advised to follow the Carnivore Diet to control and manage their health.

You will get to see different Carnivore Diet recipes, which can be used to cook different and various kinds of foods for your pleasure, taste, and satisfaction.

Popularly known as the all meat diet, the Carnivore Diet basically entails almost nothing else apart from meat irrespective of the meal or day.

Chapter 1: Story of the carnivore diet

This type of diet has been used since time immemorial by different communities around the world. Some of the infamous carnivore consumers include Mongolian nomads who solely relied on meat and dairy products.

So did Gaucho Brazilians Maasai from East Africa, Russian, Arctic, Chukotka, etc. In a recent research within the remnants of the communities relying on animal-only diet, it was discovered that half of their caloric intake mainly originated from animal fats and protein. That notwithstanding, heart disease cases were significantly lower compared to those of Caucasian Americans.

The Story of Two Cities

When we are looking at where the plants grow, we begin to see who eats plants and who does not. There are many different ways to look at what we eat and why based on what city we live in. For example, consider the Asian diet versus the African diet and how similar they are even with different biomes.

Then consider the North Pole versus the equator and how lush the equator is and how desolate the pole is. Diets will be very diverse under these conditions.

Fish versus beef applies to the coast versus the plains. Locations that have dairy have various different health issues from cities of old that had no dairy. The conundrum is that in today's society, there are all types of food almost everywhere.

The two cities or cultures we are going to compare are the Arctic people and the East African headsman.

The Arctic People

They lived in the northernmost parts of Alaska, Russia, Greenland, and Canada. Their diet begun changing around the late 1800s when the trade routes began giving them a way to access European foods like flour, sugar, and other dairy products. Before that, their meals primarily consisted of animal products and fats.

The East African Headsmen

They include the Samburu, Maasai, and Rendile peoples. They lived in East Africa around the area that is now Kenya and Tanzania along the equator. In their tradition, the males between 14 years and 28 years were warriors. The warriors ate only animal products, meat, and milk.

The two groups were subject to medical investigations several decades ago. From the investigations, numerous information was recorded about their diet and health when looking at meat and heart diseases

The remote region of Point Hope, Alaska, was subject to investigation. This was an isolated region in which the mostly meat diet was still being consumed. The research study was published in 1977. The inhabitants of this region represent one of the few remnants of the Eskimos. Their culture was composed of whale, seal, and walrus hunting.

The Diet Analysis of the Eskimos

The average daily intake of calories was approximated to 3,000 kcal per person. Only 15% to 20% of the rest of the calories were accounted for from carbohydrates. The largest part of the carbohydrates was in the form of glycogen or animal starch from the consumed meat. The average adult ingested less than 3 grams per day of sucrose. This was primarily from coffee and sweetened tea. Grain products were very rare.

From the research, it was found out that heart disease incidents among the residents of this region were ten times lower compared to the general population of the United States. The rare cases of heart diseases among the Eskimos have been repeatedly noted. Rabin Witch, while discussing the constitution of all Eskimos and that heart diseases were rare among them, said this was not the case with those he examined in the Eastern Arctic of Canada through which contact with the white man's culture had influenced their diet.

It is in the most northern parts of the region where people were still consuming pure traditional foods that this lack of heart issue was almost nonexistent. In the case of a pure meat Eskimo diet, there was no evidence of arteriosclerosis. The total cholesterol in the serum of these people was also lower.

For the pastoral African nomads, cardiac problems were unknown among the male Maasai warriors who ate solely animal foods. These people lived well into their 60s. From the nomads, 600 Maasai men were examined. Among them, more than half of their number were above 40 years old. The results of the research were that only one man out of the 600 had ever experienced heart problems. The researchers carried out further investigation.

They examined 50 more Maasai men who had dropped dead in various circumstances. No case of heart attack was recorded for all 50 men. Fatty and cholesterol deposits were found in the arteries of those who were being examined, but the deposits were not enough to cause artery blockages.

The Diet Analysis of the Maasai Men Versus Current Americans.

In estimation, these Maasai men received 66% of their daily calories from animal fats. They ate about 300 grams of fat and 600 milligrams of cholesterol in a day. According to the consumption of the Americans at the same time, an American person was recommended to eat 20% to 35% of fats and below 300 grams of cholesterol per day. The Maasai people were consuming far more fats and cholesterol compared to what the Americans were advised to eat.

And yet they had less overall health issues.

Meat and Blood Pressure

The Inuit are a group that lived in Greenland. They were raised on a diet rich in meat, fish and animal fat, and low in fruits, vegetables, whole grain, and dairy products. In the 1980s and 1990s they immigrated to Denmark. In the process of their immigration, they changed their diet. They started eating the way the Danish people ate. The Inuit people added more dairy products and plant foods to their menu while they reduced their animal intake.

According to the advice we are given by public health officials; the Inuit people were supposed to become healthier after adopting the Danish people's diet. However, research that was carried out showed that those Inuit people who went to Denmark and who had changed their diet had much higher blood pressure than those who remained behind.

We have the slight benefit of the doubt since the researchers did not investigate junk food intake or the pressures of migrating from nomad to city life. It is not known whether the Inuit people in Denmark ate more refined carbohydrates, salt, or other chemicals. What is important to note is that eating more fruits and vegetables and less meat did not improve or protect the health of the immigrants, at least not in the matters of their blood pressure.

This rings true even with the Maasai of East Africa; their blood pressure averaged 120/80 among the males between the ages of 14 years to 55 years. Only 1% of men had high blood pressure. For the Samburu community, their blood pressure levels averaged 112/70.

Chapter 2: Science's influence of the Carnivore Diet on the human body

How Does the Carnivore Diet Work?

Before continuing further, I want to throw a disclaimer out there. I am not a doctor, so I won't go into all the nitty gritty of everything. This is because what has worked for me may not work for you. All I can do is try to be as succinct as possible in outlining my reasoning.

Unlike the healthy living "gurus" and "reverends" who will quote outdated studies, I am of the opinion that meat sourced from ruminants features a myriad number of micronutrients, so the idea that a meat-only diet can lead to nutritional deficiency may come out a bit overblown.

Carnivores have a minimalistic digestive tract which is why they are more suited to eat meat diets. But what about omnivorous human beings? How is such a diet viable?

According to many scientific types of research, a human body requires a certain amount of proteins, vitamins, fats, and minerals to optimally operate. From a nutritional standpoint, an all-meat diet can cover all your nutritional needs even without incorporating plants into your diet. However, this doesn't imply plants aren't important. It merely means even a monotonous meat diet is still a worthy option.

I have personally been able to experience weight loss, seen reduced digestive issues, attained clearer thinking, and gotten the flexibility to eat the food I enjoy.

Carnivore Diet Food List

As earlier indicated, a carnivore diet strictly features animal food. Here are few examples of ratified carnivore diet foods.

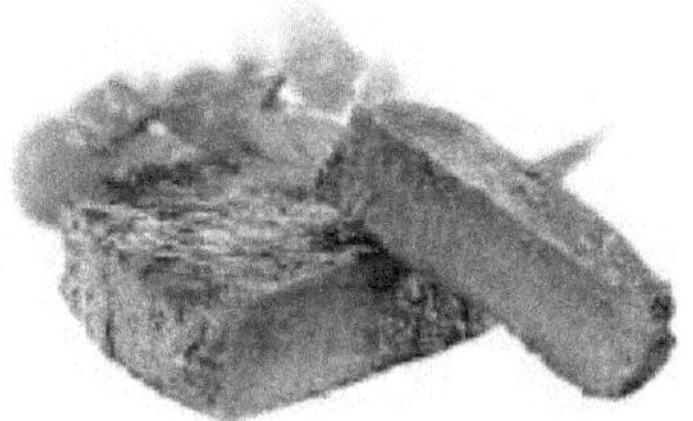

Meat-- Red meat, steak, or burgers generally form the largest catalog of the Carnivore Diet. Since you won't be indulging in any plant foods or carbs, the fatty meat cuts are the best.

Additionally, organ meats, poultry, and processed meat products in your diet also work great.

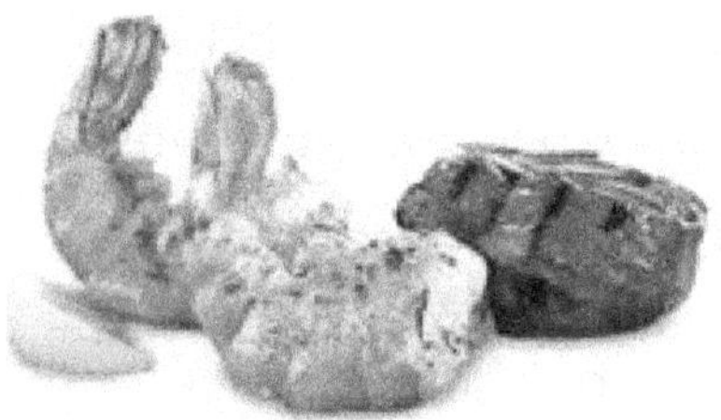

Fish -- Although any type of fish is okay, salmons and sardines are the smartest choices as they have fatty tissues.

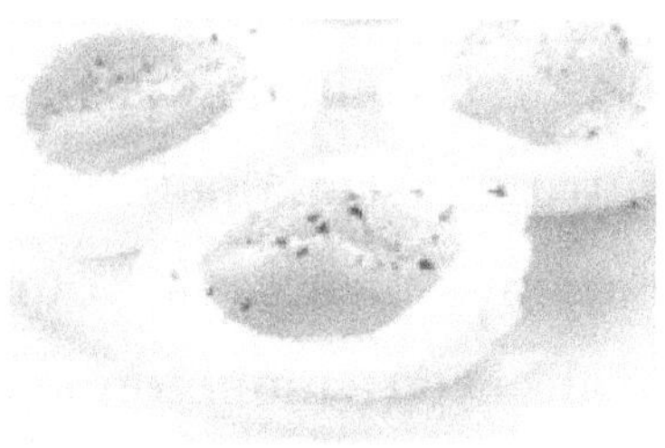

Whole Eggs -- In an egg, you should try eating only the yolks. This is because they are the most nutritious part of an egg.

Chicken eggs, goose eggs, duck eggs are allowed.

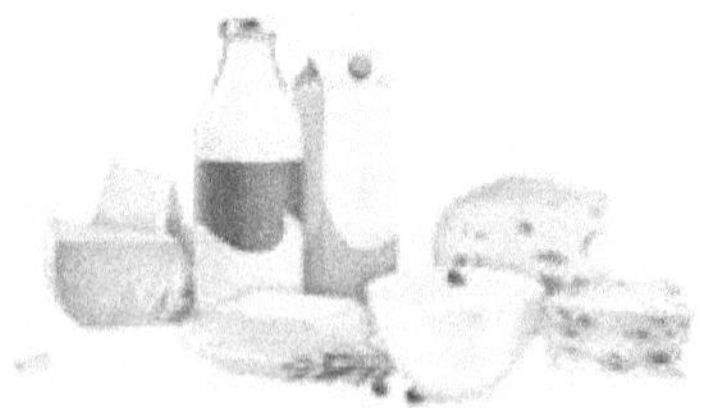

Dairy -- Although they don't fall into the category of meats; milk, butter, cheese, and yogurt are technically admissible carnivore diet elements. Many carnivore enthusiasts limit them though due to the high doses of lactose in some of these products.

Bone Marrow

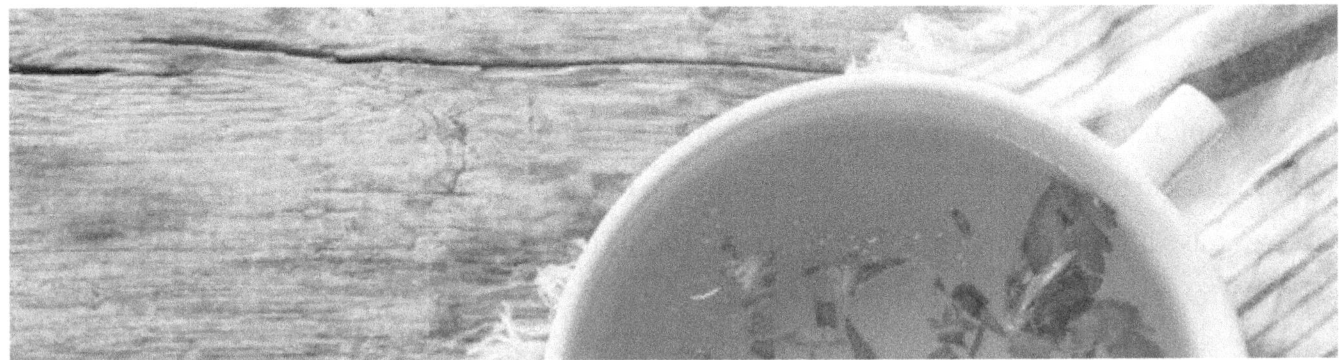

If you have been thinking that bone marrow is too fatty to be consumed, then you better think again. It's another cornerstone of the Carnivore Diet, especially when whipped in bone marrow broth.

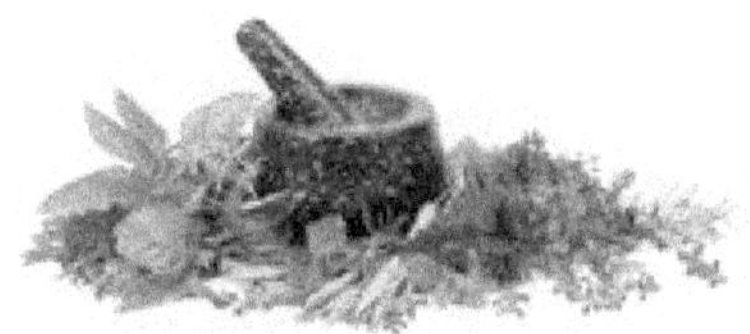

Condiments -- Just because you are consuming a Carnivore Diet, it doesn't mean your food should be stale. Since condiments such as salsa, horseradish, and mustard don't technically qualify, salt and pepper are great allies as they are considered sugar-free condiments even though they originate from plants.

Inadmissible Foods in a Carnivore Diet

As a carnivore dieter, you will have to do away with all the plant-based proteins. Packaged meat is also not recommended as it sometimes features additives which can be harmful in the long run.

Types of Carnivore Diet Drinks

The type of drinks you need to consume is entirely depended on how strict and committed you are to your carnivorous journey. As a general rule of thumb, water is the drink of choice for the first 30 days after commencing the Carnivore Diet. This could be your regular tap water, spring water, mineral water, or even filtered water.

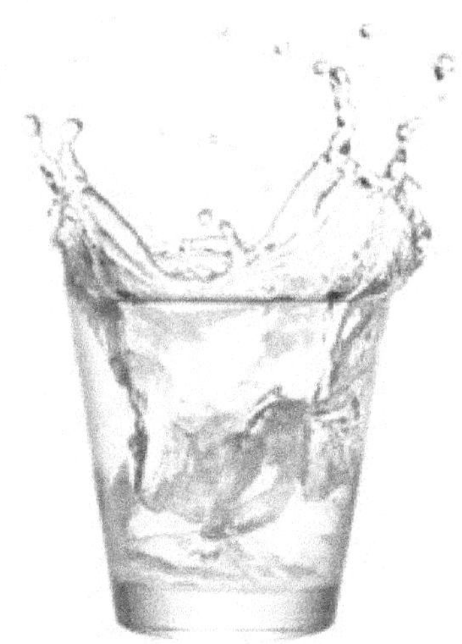

As an added requirement Dr. James Di Nicolantonio, author of *Salt Fix*, recommends adding a small pinch of salt to your water as it helps generate extra electrolytes, which help you avert any potential issues.

Carnivore Diet Benefits

Here, I would like to float another disclaimer: This e-book is based on personal experiences and a few types of research to underwrite the information. For these reasons, it shouldn't be substituted for a qualified medical opinion. Be sure to consult your doctor before venturing into any new diet.

Now to the main topic, what are the benefits of carnivore diets? Although the idea of solely eating meat may sound like a big nightmare, there are some few benefits you can reap from this diet. They include:

Weight Loss-- Albeit it would be unconventional to think that an all-meat diet would help you lose weight, the limited carbs intake lowers your blood sugar; hence your body is highly unlikely to store calories in the form of body fats. Despite the highly restricted food list that comes with carnivore diets, the proteins and fats in the food have satiating nutrients, meaning you can only eat when you are truly hungry.

Lower Inflammation-- Fat-rich foods and vegan diets promote inflammation, which can be compared to that of smoking. Although true, a recent research has indicated that a high-fat, low-carb diet can reduce systemic inflammation, which helps improve cardiovascular health.

Figure this, your liver manufactures C-reactive proteins to counter inflammation. By simply doing away with plant foods, you can significantly reduce this inflammation. Lower inflammation translates into less achy joints.

Higher Testosterone -- Carnivore diets have high-fat content, which helps boost testosterone levels. In fact, a recent study by the American Journal of Clinical Nutrition has shown individuals who committed to a high-fat, low-fiber diet for 2 ½ months showed a 13% increase in total testosterone levels compared to those that consumed low fat and high fiber. I can attest to that, as well as my testosterone levels have seen an almost 21% jump from 494 ng/dL to 570.

Reduced Digestive Problems-- Growing up, you may have been fed countless servings of dried beans and other legumes to increase the fiber levels in your body. However, the Carnivore Diet is of a different opinion and may just prove science wrong.

Increased Mental Alertness --Based on my own experience, my level of alertness and focus has certainly increased. However, I must say you may experience swings as your body tries to reconfigure how to continue operating without carbs. You may feel less energetic, experience sleeping difficulties or even get bad breath, which is something you can easily weather through.

Who Can Follow the Carnivore Diet?

Generally speaking, anybody can follow an animal-based diet. However, before you decide whether you can succeed in this journey, there are a few things I need to mention.

A human body is designed to make a smooth transition between two opposing states: The "fed" state and the "fasted" state.

Basically, the fed state means insulin levels are high, thus prompting the body to store excess energy in form of calories in the fat cells. In simple terms, the burning of calories is brought to a grinding halt with the body burning glucose collected from the last meal.

On the other hand, fasted state means insulin levels are low, which arouses growth hormones and glucagon. In this distressing state, the body is prompted to mobilize the stored body fat and convert it into energy.

Unfortunately, this is just an ideal picture. In reality, most of us spend less time fasting. This translates into our body cells spending less time mobilizing and burning the stored body fats. Eventually insulin levels rise, thus prompting the body to inhibit the burning of stored body fat, while choosing to rely on glucose.

With time, this prolonged exposure to excessive insulin prompts the body to develop 'insulin resistance,' which is the culprit behind 'Metabolic Syndrome.

Metabolic syndrome is the culprit behind elevated glucose levels, low HDL, and high triglycerides, all of which contribute to diseases like type-2 diabetes.

Although this situation is dangerous, there are multiple ways to successfully get through metabolic syndrome by becoming fat adapted and improving your body's ability to fuel itself using the stored body fat as opposed to using glucose.

This process of up-regulating the fat-burning pathway works albeit it's time-consuming and requires practice. It requires improvement of insulin sensitivity, which then lowers insulin and elevates the fat mobilization process.

As indicated, there are multiple ways of improving fat loss and a zero carb diet is one of them. These types of food have more fats and less glucose, meaning your body burns fats even when in the fed state rather than burning glucose.

The Carnivore Diet is a higher version of the keto diet, and as the name suggests, it has to do with eating animal foods only. You can eat all meat, including poultry, beef, fish, meat from organs—such as liver and kidneys—and, if you feel adventurous, the intestines and the brain. Furthermore, the meat can only be flavored with a little salt and pepper, no other seasonings are allowed.

And while some variants in the carnivorous diet accommodate for full-fat milk, the most intense practitioners totally ignore dairy. While this sounds (and is) extreme, carnivorous diet advocates saying that eating only meat helps with many health conditions, such as fatigue, obesity, and digestive health.

The drawback of the Carnivore Diet is that it is only meat, which ensures an amount of macronutrients and carbohydrates are completely missing from the diet. Carbohydrates are essential for the body to work properly. These are the food sources of the primary fuel (glucose) used by the brain and the functioning muscles which provide nutrients that are almost nonexistent in meat, such as protein, vitamins C and K, and folic acid. And while evolving science is heating up discussions regarding dietary fats, the diet of only meat, especially meat high in saturated fat, can have a negative effect on cardiovascular health.

If the supposed benefits of a carnivorous diet seem too good to be true, that's because they are. The truth is that a well-balanced diet of meat, fruit, vegetables, legumes, dairy and whole grain can make you healthier. If you discover that nutritional advice from social media leaves you confused and unsure about the type of food to eat, talk to a registered dietitian in your area to enable you to understand the details better. If you still desire to try the Carnivore Diet, you may fill half of your plate with non-starchy vegetables, such as spinach and broccoli, to add the vital nutrients missing from the meat.

Then one more thing — carnivorous diet advocates say this is how we should eat because it's how our ancestors used to live, but that's not entirely true. Early humans ate what was readily available. If you lived in a cold climate with only seafood, you would have eaten seafood. But if you stayed in a lush jungle with a variety of fruits and vegetables, then your diet was full of fruit and vegetables (and maybe bugs). As in the past and today, there is not just one diet humans can choose to follow.

The Carnivore Diet is a restricted diet that contains only beef, fish and other animal foods such as eggs and certain dairy products.

It excludes all other foods, including fruit, vegetables, legumes, grains, nuts and seeds.

The advocates also advise that milk consumption be avoided or limited to items poor in lactose — sugar is present in milk and dairy products — such as butter and hard cheese.

The Carnivore Diet research comes from the controversial belief that human ancestral populations have eaten mostly meat and fish and that high-carb diets are responsible for today's high rates of chronic disease.

Chapter 3: What is right what is wrong

Because of the highly restrained nature and total removal of most food groups, there are a lot of issues related to the Carnivore Diet.

The problems or issues associated with the Carnivore Diet include:

It is high in fat, cholesterol, saturated fats and sodium since the Carnivore Diet includes mainly animal foods. Saturated fat might increase your LDL (bad) cholesterol, which might raise the risk of a person having heart disease.

Meanwhile, the latest studies have proven that the high intake of saturated fat and cholesterol are not highly related to an increased risk of heart disease, as was formerly thought.

However, taking in high amounts of saturated fat on the Carnivore Diet might be of worry. No study has proven the consequences of eating animal foods only.

And that means the effects of eating high cholesterol and fats are not identified and known by anyone.

Likewise, some processed portions of meat, particularly breakfast meats and bacon, also include high amounts of sodium.

Whenever you consume a lot of these foods associated with the Carnivore Diet, it will result in too much sodium intake, which has been related to a high risk of kidney disease, high blood pressure and other adverse health issues.

Intake of processed meat also relates to increased rates of particular kinds of cancer, which includes of rectal and colon cancer.

Might Lack some micronutrients and beneficial plant compounds

The Carnivore Diet removes highly nourishing foods like vegetables, legumes, fruits as well as grains, which include beneficial minerals and vitamins.

While meat can be nourishing and offers micronutrients, it ought not to be the only part of your diet. A restrained diet, such as the Carnivore Diet might result in deficiencies in a few nutrients and overconsumption of other kinds.

The Carnivore Diet, which is rich in animal-based foods, has been related to a lesser risk of some chronic situations such as cancers, heart disease, Alzheimer's, and diabetes.

It is not only because of the high fiber, vitamin, and mineral substance of plant foods, but also includes their beneficial antioxidants and other compounds.

The Carnivore Dies does not include these stated compounds and are not concerning any long term health gains.

Does not provide fiber - Fiber is known to be a non-digestible carb that encourages gut health and healthy bowel progress and is only seen in plant foods.

The Carnivore Diet includes no fiber at all, which might result in constipation in some individuals.

Also, fiber is unbelievably necessary for the right stability of bacteria in your gut.

Meanwhile, suboptimal gut health can result in some problems and might even be related to destabilized immunity and colon cancer.

Research conducted revealed that 17 obese were on a high-protein and low carb-diet, which reduced their levels of compounds that assist in guarding against colon cancer, measuring up to high-protein and moderate-carb diets.

Generally, following the Carnivore Diet might damage your gut health.

Carnivore Diet may not be the best option for a few populations

The Carnivore Diet might have issues for some communities. For instance, the people who must reduce their protein intake and those who have chronic kidney disease are not advised to follow the Carnivore Diet.

Furthermore, those who are sensitive to cholesterol in foods should be careful about eating meals high in cholesterol.

Also, some populations with unique nutrient requirements would probably not meet them while they are on the Carnivore Diet. It may include women who are breastfeeding or pregnant. People who are anxious about food or find it difficult to restrain their eating should look away from the Carnivore Diet.

Advantage/Disadvantage of the Carnivore Diet

Disadvantages of the Carnivore Diet
One of the disadvantages of an all meat diet is it can harm your health instead of improving it if you don't eat meat that is of good quality. The cheaper industrially processed meats are usually full of many preservatives, residues and chemicals. These animals are fed low quality food filled with toxins like pesticides, GMOs, antibiotics, etc. which then go into their body.

You will thus be indirectly eating all these from the low-quality meat as well. This is why it is important to find meat from animals raised in pastures, grass-fed or fed organic food. This will ensure the animals were healthy, and so therefore, is the meat. This factor is essential when you follow a meat-based diet.

Since meat contains a lot of saturated fat and cholesterol, you will get a lot of it in your diet on a regular basis. This might be a disadvantage. The trans-fat from this diet might also prompt the liver to produce more cholesterol than required. This is why you need to control the amount of fatty meat you consume regularly.

Another drawback is the high amount of sodium found in processed meat or salt-cured meat. Excessive consumption of sodium can escalate the risk of heart diseases or strokes and even be a problem for kidney function. This is why it is recommended to avoid processed meat like salami, jerky or ham in order to avoid the excess sodium. Fresh meat will have much lower levels of sodium and is not a cause for concern.

If you consider the cost factor, it is true that a meat diet is more expensive than a plant-based diet. The diet can be quite expensive if you are providing it not just for yourself but your entire family. Buying meat is expensive on a daily basis, especially if you want the good quality kind. Unless you have your own farm animals or can somehow process the meat yourself, you should be prepared to increase expenditure on food in your budget. One tip that will help is buying in bulk as it usually reduces the cost.

Advantages of the Carnivore Diet
The advantage of this diet is that it is fairly simple. It saves you a lot of time and energy since your ingredients and cooking process are both simplified. You won't just see improvement in your health, but also notice you spend a lot less of your day in the kitchen preparing food. Most of the cutting, processing, and cooking involved in your usual day are removed when you follow the Carnivore Diet.

The Carnivore Diet is a great source of protein for the body. Protein is essential for maintaining many processes in the body to keep it healthy. This is why it is considered a building block of life. Since you will only be eating meat, you have a constant source of good protein for your body. Even a small amount of meat is densely packed with protein and will make up for the recommended daily allowance for a person.

You will also be getting all the essential amino acids required by your body. Nine amino acids exist that cannot be made by the body even though they are essential for health. The proteins in meat contain amino acids and actually have all nine of them. This is why animal meat is considered a complete source of protein and supplements the body with these essential amino acids through the diet. In order for maintaining healthy bones, muscle and skin, these amino acids need to be provided regularly.

You will also be getting a good source of B-complex vitamins such as niacin, riboflavin, thiamine and vitamin B12. Meat contains all of these and thus helps to maintain energy levels and contributes to growth. These vitamins also help with better iron absorption. Meat will also provide other minerals such as zinc and selenium to your body.

Another advantage is this diet has helped a lot of people overcome some chronic illnesses, which they could not otherwise treat. This includes autoimmune diseases and even includes Lyme disease. When other treatments and even a good doctor's protocol failed, this diet helped a lot of people get healthier on a purely meat-based diet.

The Effect of the Carnivore Diet on Cholesterol

A common misconception is that eating meat, butter or even eggs is one of the main causes of high levels of bad cholesterol. You will hear a lot of so-called weight gurus telling you to stop eating any of these if you want to lose weight or improve your health. You probably doubt the validity of us saying a diet rich in these foods won't affect your health in any way and especially in terms of alcohol. It might make you feel like we are saying that eating a lot of junk food won't make you fat. But on an honest note, the two are in no way similar.

Cholesterol itself has many misconceptions associated with it. In this section, we will try and explain more about how your diet will affect your cholesterol levels and if you should be worried or not. But before you do this, you have to keep an open mind and let go of the misconceptions you already have. Only then will you understand how it works and why the Carnivore Diet is healthy for you.

Most of what we know about cholesterol is not true and is just based on unreasonable statements made by certain people who themselves don't understand any better. Cholesterol is a wax-like substance produced by humans and animals. No other living form produces cholesterol; so, all plant sources are free of it. A lot of research has shown people with clogged arteries are more likely to suffer from cardiovascular health issues. There is a direct link between the arteries and the heart, and it affects your health.

The more clogged your arteries are, the higher your chances of suffering from a stroke or cardiac arrest. From this research, they concluded cholesterol was to blame for heart issues since it was what clogged the arteries. This is why people were told if they ate foods rich in cholesterol, it would increase levels in their body and thus cause heart ailments. Naturally, people started demonizing red meat, butter, eggs and such cholesterol rich food.

However, do high cholesterol foods affect the levels in your body? The answer is no because your body already knows how to control levels of cholesterol. Since the human body itself produces cholesterol, it has its mechanism to maintain healthy levels in the body. It works like a feedback mechanism where the body stops producing cholesterol when it notices there are high levels of it already. Similarly, if the level of cholesterol decreases, the body produces more of it.

What you need to understand is cholesterol is not all bad. It has its classification of good cholesterol and bad cholesterol. This is what you need to pay attention to. Cholesterol exists as a fat molecule that isn't soluble like salt or sugar. This is why it needs a medium to travel through the body since it will not dissolve in the blood itself.

The medium used by cholesterol molecules is lipoproteins. They are a mixed molecule group, which contain both protein and fat. The main function of lipoproteins is cholesterol transport to organs or cells when required. Among lipoproteins, there is a classification of two types that are responsible for this cholesterol transport. One is high-density lipoprotein or HDL, and the other is low-density lipoprotein or LDL. Although the HDL and LDL can't technically be called cholesterol, they are known as good and bad cholesterol.

The function of HDL molecules is to transport cholesterol from different parts of your body to your liver. In the liver, it is either removed or reused for the body. The LDL molecules transport cholesterol from the liver to the rest of the body. If the level of HDL or good cholesterol is high in your body, you risk of cardiovascular diseases is lower. To increase the level of HDL, your diet should be rich in natural dietary fibers. This is why a low carbohydrate diet has a positive effect by increasing HDL levels.

On the other hand, the LDL level should not be high, and this is why it is called bad cholesterol; however, it is just a low-density lipoprotein and not actual cholesterol. The LDL itself is responsible for transporting cholesterol, and when the level of this is high, more cholesterol is taken to the liver. Increased LDL levels are responsible for the higher risk of heart ailments.

The smaller LDL particles further contribute to this negative impact. When you consume a low carb diet, it helps to turn these into larger molecules and also causes a reduction of LDL in the blood. By now you can understand that a dietary fat-rich diet will not cause issues in cholesterol. This kind of diet facilitates a more balanced cholesterol level in the body.

Just like cholesterol, people are also wary of triglyceride levels. But most of the fears related to triglycerides are quite baseless. Triglycerides are a type of fat most commonly found in food. They help to provide fuel for the body. The only difference is they are used as fuel storage for the future and not for immediate use by the body.

When your body is breaking down sugars to use for energy, some of it is stored in cells as triglycerides. The more the body deals with carbohydrates, the more insulin it produces. Too much insulin will cause problems with blood sugar in the body, and this will then increase the stored triglyceride levels. So, it is the fats that you need to worry about. Eating a diet low in carbs will help to prevent any such problems. This is why the Carnivore Diet eliminates carbs and helps to maintain good health.

Don't let myths and misconceptions about cholesterol and triglycerides mislead you. It is important to learn the scientific reasoning behind something before believing what is told in general. A half-truth is equal to a lie and can be harmful. When you learn more about something, it helps you understand it better.

This is why we are making an effort to explain the details of the Carnivore Diet and its effect on the body to you. This book is not just some blank guide that tells you to do this and that while making false claims. We are here to help you understand how things work in your body and why we recommend this particular diet to help you lose unwanted weight, get lean and stay healthy for a long time.

Potential challenges and risks

Nutrient Deficiencies

Now that we have put in place some of the mechanisms involved, the big question is: Can the Carnivore Diet be considered safe enough?

The obvious answer is we really don't know, because long-term experiments have not monitored broad groups of individuals on carnivorous diets for any significant length of time. One of my main concerns is the scarcity of a variety of nutrients essential for nutrition.

Four micronutrients are extremely difficult to obtain on a meat-only diet. Based on the standard carnivorous diet and dietary guide intakes (DRIs) developed by the Institute of Medicine, these include:

Vitamin C: An antioxidant which enhances immune cell function and is essential for promoting collagen synthesis.

Vitamin E: An antioxidant that prevents the oxidation of lipids and lipoproteins.

Vitamin K2: A fat-soluble vitamin which decreases the calcification of blood vs. Nevertheless, if you don't like animal food, the number of potential micronutrient deficiencies increases significantly.

Vitamin A: Fat-soluble vitamin essential for proper vision and immune defenses.

Folate: B vitamin critical for cell growth, digestion, and methylation.

Manganese: A trace mineral required for the proper functioning of the nervous system, collagen production and oxidative stress safety.

Magnesium: A mineral which helps more than 300 biochemical reactions in the body. It helps to maintain normal nerve and muscle function.

Some carnivores say the food standards for the general population actually do not extend to them. Anecdotally, I hear of a few people who have been consuming carnivorous diets for three or more years without any clear signs of nutrient deficiencies.

Still, we lack the details. Currently, the DRIs are the option we have to get away from, and I don't believe we have enough evidence to say confidently that this program has no chance of causing nutrient deficiencies in the general population.

Should we aim higher than the recommended daily intake?

Even if the Carnivore Diet is sufficient to prevent a full deficit, we should also find the metabolic reserve. The caloric capacity is the strength of cells, tissues and organ systems to tolerate frequent shifts in physiological needs. In other terms, there is enough food in the tank to cope with a big stressor, illness, or damage to the climate. Thus, if an all-meat diet is able to meet the recommended intake of nutrients, it may still not be sufficient for optimal health.

Certain potential side effects of an all-meat diet that lacks beneficial phytonutrients which help your nutrition phytonutrients are chemicals generated by plants to defend against environmental risks, such as insect and disease assaults. They can also have major health benefits. Curcumin, beta-carotene, quercetin and resveratrol are examples of popular phytonutrients.

Some Carnivore Diet advocates say phytonutrients are toxic to humans and that it is best to remove them entirely from our food. Nevertheless, many of these 'toxins' function as acute stressors that actually make us stronger through a process called hormesis.

It could shortchange your liver (if you're consuming lean meat). When you don't eat enough carbohydrates and fat, your liver can make protein glucose through a process called gluconeogenesis. The process creates nitrogenous waste, which must be transformed into urea and disposed of through the kidneys.

The Effects of the Carnivore Diet on Digestion

Your digestive system plays a major role in your body. Your diet has a major impact on your digestion in turn. This is why it is important to pay due heed to the effects of the various foods you eat on your digestion. Every system in your body is interlinked, and a problem with one will also cause health issues in other regards. This section will help you understand the effect of the Carnivore Diet on the digestive system.

Every healthy gut has a couple of kilograms of microbes in it. These include nearly a thousand different species of bacteria, and the health of these microbes will affect your digestive health. Bacteria are not always bad. The ones that are naturally in your stomach aid in the digestive process and are essential for good gut health. They help your body to absorb nutrients from the food that is being digested.

The small intestine and stomach cannot ingest every type of food. At this point, the microbes come in and do it for them. This is why it is important to support good microbe health in your gut. The foods you eat will determine this. Some foods will aid in this and others will cause a negative reaction.

Processed foods and sugar are not good for your digestive system. This is why the Carnivore Diet requires you to eliminate any such foods and focus on healthy fat and meat-based food. Sugars and processed foods will cause undesirable bacteria to grow in your gut. This will cause an imbalance in a healthy microbiome system in your gut.

Your digestive system is affected, and food is not digested optimally. The good bacteria in your gut are harmed by all the sugars, artificial sweeteners and ingredients in processed food. This is why they need to be eliminated if you want the probiotic bacteria to thrive in your digestive system while eliminating harmful bacteria.

A leaky gut can be another problem in an unhealthy digestive system. The Carnivore Diet also aids in preventing this and restoring health. In the foods you eat, not every substance is desirable for your body. The good bacteria and a healthy gut make sure these stay within the gastrointestinal tract since they act as a barrier. When your gut lining is not in a healthy condition, the barrier is also not effective.

This means the harmful substances can escape from the gastrointestinal tract and get into the bloodstream. This can be a very dangerous situation for your body. It is not just harmful bacteria that get into your bloodstream, but food particles and toxins as well. This is why it is important to pay attention to gut health so a healthy barrier is maintained.

A leaky gut will show adverse effects on various aspects of your body. This includes your skin, hormones as well as your brain. You might wonder how the carnivore diet aids in preventing this. The restriction of foods therefore plays an important role. Grains, as well as legumes, can cause weakening of the barrier. The gluten in these foods can be a major cause of autoimmune disorders.

There is a protein molecule called Zonulin that is activated by gluten from grains. This protein molecule breaks the bonds between the cells within the intestinal walls and gut lining. The lectins and phytic acids in these foods also weaken the barrier and are thus bad for gut health. These foods can also end up being a cause of leaky gut syndrome that is a very harmful digestive condition that you need to prevent.

The Carnivore Diet does not include any of these grains or legumes, so it does not harm the gut lining. The dietary fats will instead help to release proteins that will strengthen the gut by reducing inflammation.

The modern western diet is sadly lacking in terms of healthy dietary fats. People have reduced their fat intake as much as possible since they believe it is the culprit behind weight gain and other health issues. The truth is that carbohydrates are the cause and fats are healthy. These carbs should be eliminated instead, and the Carnivore Diet helps to do this. Instead, you are encouraged to eat food that has a lot of dietary fat like meat and other dairy products.

Eating grass-fed meat along with seafood will give you a regular healthy supply of omega 3 fatty acids. These are healthy and increase the diversity of the bacteria essential for proper digestion. This microbiome unit in the stomach is quite like a small ecosystem by itself and diversity is always a good way to evolve. The more your diet comprises of healthy fats, the more diverse it will be, and thus it is better for your health.

Nearly all the health problems suffered by these few generations have been caused by the unhealthy modern diet and lifestyle. The way we eat, how we live all affects us negatively and thus causes illness. The food in the modern diet is full of GMOs, pesticides, chemicals, additives, etc. and these damages your gut as a whole. When you switch to the basic way of eating followed by our ancestors, you will improve the health of the digestive system. The more processed food you eat, the worse it gets. The Carnivore Diet will help to prevent such unhealthy conditions.

If you are worried about the lack of fiber in the diet, you should not be. Most of us have been told that fiber is essential for a healthy digestive system and regular bowel movements. The carnivore diet lacks this factor; however, fiber is not as important as it is made out to be. Instead of fiber, the healthy fat in your food will help in bowel regulation. These dietary fats ease the process of waste elimination from the body.

You might notice it is less frequent than usual, but this is normal. The Carnivore Diet itself is the reason behind it. Your body just does not need to get rid of as much waste as it does in the usual diet. It is true that fiber is important for certain people due to their particular genetic makeup, but it is not necessary for everyone to consume a high fiber diet.

You must know that every system in the body is interlinked in some way or the other, so the digestive system is also linked to the brain. Your gut works as a new brain in your body. This is why people say, "Go with your gut" when you have to make some decisions. There is a lot of research that says that the gut and mind are quite connected. Your gut is strongly linked to your emotions even if you might not have thought of it before.

Have you noticed how your stomach seems to ache when you are scared or nervous or how there is a sensation like butterflies moving at times? This is why there are so many sayings related to the gut. There is scientific reasoning behind this too. The enteric nervous system or ENS is present in the gut. This ENS has control over secretions and blood flow within the gastrointestinal tract. Due to this system, you can feel what is happening in your gut. This is why the gut has a lot of control over digestion in your body.

When you experience stress, even this is connected to the functioning of your gut. Are you familiar with the fight or flight instinct? This is an instinct in humans that help them to protect themselves. This instinct is responsible for the regulation of cortisol level in your body. The body functions normally when there is no stress. But when you are experiencing stress, the body also experiences this fight or flight emotion.

The human body seems incapable of differentiating between physical and psychological stress. If you are someone who deals with chronic stress or anxiety, you are at high risk of chronic inflammation. The same way your body reacts if there is an infection, it will react in case of stress. It is important to try and alleviate such stress from your daily life if you want to prevent the damage from inflammation on your system.

Pay heed to the connection between your mind and gut. The body has a way of letting you know when it is in distress so that you can make an effort to take care of it. If you eat a healthy diet like the Carnivore Diet, it will improve your gut health and also ensure good mental health. The leaky gut syndrome we mentioned earlier could even cause mental fog, so beware of these symptoms. Improving gut health will restore mental clarity.

Chapter 4: Kitchen tools for easy preparation

Recommended Product Cooking Equipment

Here is a directory of cooking appliances and utensils. I like the bamboo slicing block from Amazon.

Good knife for slicing any kind of meat—Get a sharp knife designed to cut large chunks into smaller portions for frying. I like this Amazon Victorinox Fibrox Pro blade.

Good steak knife package—Quickly cuts through your tender steak when you're cooking. I like this kitchen knife package with an Amazon storage block and knife sharpener.

Cast iron stew or barbecue plate—Roasts the beef on the top of the stove like a pro chef. I like this Le Creuset signature iron handle stew on Amazon to prepare something.

When cooking steak, you can cook your meat as you like on a zero carb diet (Carnivore Diet).

High-end steak restaurants that value good quality food serve red meat, such as beef, medium rare and not well done. If you're not a steak lover who's meat is still pink or mildly bloody; you may notice your preferences can change over time as you eat meat every day. You're likely to start eating a mild, rare steak vs. a well-done steak.

Cook other meats (chicken, bacon, fish) to make sure they are safe to eat. For starters, from a food safety point of view, I would not eat raw chicken or raw bacon. Nonetheless, raw fish is a must try, fried salmon, tuna sashimi or new oysters.

All food that does not come from animals is excluded from the Carnivore Diet. Restricted foods include:

Vegetables: Broccoli, cauliflower, potatoes, green beans, peppers, etc.

Fruits: Strawberries, grapes, bananas, kiwis, oranges, etc.

High-lactose butter: Milk, cereal, soft cheese, etc.

Legumes: Peas, lentils, etc.

Nuts and seeds: Peanuts, pumpkin seeds, sunflower seeds, pistachios, etc.

Grain: Corn, maize, barley, quinoa, pasta, etc.

Alcohol: Beer, wine, liqueur, etc.

Sugar: Table sugar, maple syrup, brown sugar, etc.

Beverages other than water: Soda, espresso, tea, fruit, etc.

While some people use some of these foods, they are not permitted by the real Carnivore Diet.

Products not derived from animals were completely excluded, including plants, berries, high-lactose dairy products, legumes, nuts, beans, wheat, beer, coffee, tea and juices.

The primary focus should be on fatty meat, especially BEEF.

The next thing on your plan is beef, pork, chicken and fish.

Then…if you want…eggs, then low-carbon dairy products like milk, heavy whipping cream and hard cheese.

Your Beef Cuts: Steaks (ribeye, sirloin, slice, ribbed eye)

Roasts: Prime rib, duck, brisket

Ground beef: Organs if you want (though not required)

How much to eat on a carnivore diet when you're tired

Eat until you're full. Yeah, listen to your body. It has been found the majority of people had an average of two meals a day. But some may do best with three meals a day, while others do the best with one meal a day. Neither 1, 2, 3 nor 4 is better than the other.

Let your appetite guide you through it.

As your body is changing and recovering from years of deprivation, it is normal for you to consume twice as much as you have been recovered.

Feed well. Your body is starving for it.

2-4 lbs. of fatty meat per day can be used as a guide.

It is essential that you do not deliberately limit your calories or food intake or require fasting. I'm going to explain why.

Foods Not Allowed on the Carnivore Diet:

Vegetables, fruit, seeds, legumes, wheat, pasta and grains. None of these foods are allowed on the Carnivore Diet.

Protein Cooking Methods

The primary goals while cooking meat is to develop flavor, tenderness, and juiciness. Meat is a major part of the food budget while on the Carnivore Diet. So the secondary important goal is to enhance cooked yield. The end results of cooking are determined by a number of factors. Some of the factors that determine how successful the cooking will be are:

The method of cooking. Different cooking methods produce different results. For example, boiling meat will not produce the same flavor results as roasting meat.

The type of meal. Different types of meals are cooked differently, and the results differ.

The experience of the cook. The person who prepares meals matters a lot. The more talented the chef, the better the meal.

The Science of Cooking Proteins

Proteins that come from animals are mostly made up of water. The amount of time taken to cook is affected by the type of meat, cooking temperature, and cooking medium. When the meat is cooked too much or for too long, it becomes tough and dry. The yield goes down. In order to get the best out of the cooking process, one has to determine which process is the best for a specific meal. Optimizing the cooking process preserves the quality of the end product. Well-cooked meat has a low amount of moisture loss and shrinkage.

Protein in meat exists in the form of muscle fibers. Muscle fibers are held together by tendons, which is connective tissue. Tendons connect the muscle fibers to the bone structure. Fats are deposited around the muscle fibers. Inside them, there are smaller fascicles that determine the grain and tenderness of the meat. Meat from less exercised muscles appears grained and smooth in texture. Meat from the muscles that are more exercised is tough and coarse in texture.

Tender is, in most cases, used as a description of quality in meat. Various factors determine the tenderness of the meat. This included the age of the animal, the amount of marbling, the part of the animal where the cut came from, and the process of cooking them.

Tenderness does not always determine flavor. The flavor is mostly determined by the fats in an animal. Flavor and tenderness come together on the cooking process. Some cuts of the meat have more flavor than others.

The Cooking Processes

When meat and other animal proteins are raw, they appear soft and relaxed. When heat is applied, it squeezes together and pushes out moisture. The higher the cooking temperature, the more it expels moisture and become tough. But as the protein continues to cook, it regains its tenderness.

Doneness for meat and other proteins are determined by the species, the individual cuts, and the desired outcome. For smaller tender cuts of meat, you can determine doneness by touch method. In this, you exert pressure at the surface of the item. For large roasts of meat, the temperature method is used. This method is gauged with a thermometer. For tough cuts, the fork-tender method is applied. The meat is pierced with a fork; if the fork goes through the meat, most likely, the meat is done.

Choosing a Cooking Method

Several factors are considered when one wants to prepare a meal. Certain incisive factors have to be strictly checked, such as the health of the people who the meal is intended for. The number of nutrients and vitamins in the cooked meal is also a consideration. More factors include the following:

Type of meal being cooked.

Various foods are cooked using various methods. For example, chicken liver is better when fried than when boiled.

Loss of nutrients.

Nutrients are lost when a certain method of cooking is used. For example, certain nutrients that are soluble in water can be lost if the meat is boiled, and the stock is discarded.

Facilities are available.

Various facilities are necessary for different cooking methods. For instance, a roasting grill is necessary when roasting meat.

Age and health of people to eat the food.

This is a very important factor that has to be considered. For instance, children and elderly people require their food to be cooked using the most easily digestible methods like boiling and steaming.

Available time.

Some methods require a longer time than others. For instance, boiling an egg takes a longer time than frying an egg. Individuals with little time in the kitchen will most probably choose the method that is more convenient according to the time limit.

The method the cook is familiar with.

Different people prefer different methods of cooking. One person may be good at roasting, yet another may be talented with frying. The method to be used for cooking will matter on who is on duty.

Different methods of cooking produce varying results of the end product.

The flavor may also change depending on the method. But what matters most is people get to eat clean, well cooked and healthy meals.

We shall look at protein cooking methods. This will help you more in knowing how to go about the Carnivore Diet, which is about eating proteins all the time.

Tips for Protein Cooking Methods

The primary goals while cooking meat is to develop flavor, tenderness, and juiciness. Meat is a major part of the food budget while on the Carnivore Diet. So the secondary important goal is to enhance cooked yield. The end results of cooking are determined by a number of factors. Some of the factors that determine how successful the cooking will be are:

The method of cooking. Different cooking methods produce different results. For example, boiling meat will not produce the same flavor results as roasting meat.

The type of meal. Different types of meals are cooked differently, and the results differ.

The experience of the cook. The person who prepares meals matters a lot. The more talented the chef, the better the meal.

The Science of Cooking Proteins

Proteins that come from animals are mostly made up of water. The amount of time taken to cook is affected by the type of meat, cooking temperature, and cooking medium. When the meat is cooked too much or for too long, it becomes tough and dry. The yield goes down. In order to get the best out of the cooking process, one has to determine which process is the best for a specific meal. Optimizing the cooking process preserves the quality of the end product. Well-cooked meat has a low amount of moisture loss and shrinkage.

Protein in meat exists in the form of muscle fibers. Muscle fibers are held together by tendons, which is connective tissue. Tendons connect the muscle fibers to the bone structure. Fats are deposited around the muscle fibers. Inside them, there are smaller fascicles that determine the grain and tenderness of the meat. Meat from less exercised muscles appears grained and smooth in texture. Meat from the muscles that are more exercised is tough and coarse in texture.

Tender is, in most cases, used as a description of quality in meat. Various factors determine the tenderness of the meat. This included the age of the animal, the amount of marbling, the part of the animal where the cut came from, and the process of cooking them.

Tenderness does not always determine flavor. The flavor is mostly determined by the fats in an animal. Flavor and tenderness come together on the cooking process. Some cuts of the meat have more flavor than others.

The Cooking Processes

When meat and other animal proteins are raw, they appear soft and relaxed. When heat is applied, it squeezes together and pushes out moisture. The higher the cooking temperature, the more it expels moisture and become tough. But as the protein continues to cook, it regains its tenderness.

Doneness for meat and other proteins are determined by the species, the individual cuts, and the desired outcome. For smaller tender cuts of meat, you can determine doneness by touch method. In this, you exert pressure at the surface of the item. For large roasts of meat, the temperature method is used. This method is gauged with a thermometer. For tough cuts, the fork-tender method is applied. The meat is pierced with a fork; if the fork goes through the meat, most likely, the meat is done.

Choosing a Cooking Method

Several factors are considered when one wants to prepare a meal. Certain incisive factors have to be strictly checked, such as the health of the people who the meal is intended for. The number of nutrients and vitamins in the cooked meal is also a consideration. More factors include the following:

Type of meal being cooked.

Various foods are cooked using various methods. For example, chicken liver is better when fried than when boiled.

Loss of nutrients.

Nutrients are lost when a certain method of cooking is used. For example, certain nutrients that are soluble in water can be lost if the meat is boiled, and the stock is discarded.

Facilities are available.

Various facilities are necessary for different cooking methods. For instance, a roasting grill is necessary when roasting meat.

Age and health of people to eat the food.

This is a very important factor that has to be considered. For instance, children and elderly people require their food to be cooked using the most easily digestible methods like boiling and steaming.

Available time.

Some methods require a longer time than others. For instance, boiling an egg takes a longer time than frying an egg. Individuals with little time in the kitchen will most probably choose the method that is more convenient according to the time limit.

The method the cook is familiar with.

Different people prefer different methods of cooking. One person may be good at roasting, yet another may be talented with frying. The method to be used for cooking will matter on who is on duty.

Different methods of cooking produce varying results of the end product.

The flavor may also change depending on the method. But what matters most is people get to eat clean, well cooked and healthy meals.

We shall look at protein cooking methods. This will help you more in knowing how to go about the Carnivore Diet, which is about eating proteins all the time.

Tips for Protein Cooking Methods

Cooking is the art of making food ready for easier ingestion using heat. Cooking methods and ingredients differ across the world, depending on diverse environments, cultures, economies, and trends. Also, cooking techniques rely on one's skills and training.

When cooking your food, ensure every meal that you eat has a high protein content. Proteins help in building your muscles, hormones, skin, and different body organs. The recommended daily protein intakes differ from each gender. For example, men should get 56 grams of proteins daily, while women should get 46 grams of proteins every day.

Tips and Tricks While Cooking Protein Dishes

1. Eggs

Whole eggs are possibly the most nutritious foods on Earth. They contain minerals, vitamins, brain nutrients, and healthy fats. A white egg protein content consists of 35 percent calories. The delicious and extremely versatile source of protein can be cooked in different ways and are easy to combine with other parts of the Carnivore Diet.

A well-cooked egg is free from any dangerous bacteria, making them safe for consumption. Below are the ordinary egg cooking methods.

Poaching Method

Poached eggs are chilled in slightly cold water. The eggs are then cracked into a pot of simmering water between 71-82 degrees Celsius and then prepared for 2.5-3 minutes.

A spoon or wire scoop is used to remove them from the simmering water.

Boiled Method

It is recommended to put your hard-boiled eggs into ice water. This will separate the shell from the white.

Frying Method

When frying an egg, you crack it into a hot pan containing a thin layer of cooking oil or, in the case of the carnivore diet, fat. With the modern invention of Teflon, it is possible to avoid oil altogether. You can opt to prepare the eggs by frying one side (sunny side up), or you can fry the egg on both sides (over easy).

2. Beef

Beef is a rich source of protein. There are massive varieties of cooking techniques you can use to prepare each beef cut for a delicious and nutritious meal. Some of the cooking methods include the following:

Grilling

Grilling is a cooking technique that uses low, medium, or high heat. The best steaks for grilling include rib eye, T-bones, porterhouse, and strip steaks.

Grilling is considered the healthiest cooking alternative to flying since instead of cooking in oil or fat, the fat drips away from the meat.

To grill your meat, you need a rack, grill, coals, and elongated tongs.

Marinating

Marinating is rare for the carnivore diet. The best marinade is one of water and meat stock from a previous meal. Bones and marrow left to simmer will make an excellent marinade.

A strict carnivore diet does not allow for spice here. Experimentation with the limited content of this diet is up to the user.

Smoking Method

The smoking method is a way of cooking meat over a fire. Chips of wood are added to the fire to give your meat a smoky flavor. The most popular meats for smoking include pork shoulders, briskets, and ribs. You can also smoke lamb legs, fish, or chicken. To smoke your beef, you need a smoke holding container and a source of smoke.

Other than hardwood, you can use a bought smoker that uses fuel or electricity. However, the type of smoker that will work for you will depend on various factors such as space, fuel to use, and your budget. Smokers range in sizes of large box smokers to small drum smokers. If you opt to use hardwood, it is crucial to soak the wood in water for about one hour. Wet wood will lasts longer compared to fresh woods.

The smoking method requires excellent temperature control. The best range for smoking meat is 200 to 220 degrees Fahrenheit. For better meat cooking results, you need to cook your meat to an internal temperature of 145 degrees for beef and 165 degrees for chicken. However, meat smoking is a long process and can easily dry out completely. Temperature control is essential.

3. Fish

Fish is a rich source of protein. There are different ways of cooking fresh fish for it to turn delicious and moist. Some of the cooking methods include the following:

Poaching Method

Poaching is an excellent method of cooking all seafood. The cooking technique keeps your fish moist without masking the delicate fish flavor. To poach your fish, use something like chicken stock. The following procedures are the best when poaching your fish for tasty food.

Ensure all the pieces of fish are well spread on a big pan lying flat.

Brush the fish in fat from another animal or fish.

Ensure the liquified meat fat is just below the boiling point.

In case you see any bubbles developing from the pan's bottom, the liquid is too hot hence you should let it slightly cool.

The best temperatures for poaching should not exceed 180 degrees Fahrenheit.

Gently simmer until the fish flakes can be comfortably picked using a fork.

Grilling Method

Grilling is best for small fish fillets such as sardines and mackerel. The cooking technique gives a beautiful and crisp skin. To start, use fat to brush the fillets. Lay the fillets on an oiled baking sheet, skin-side up, and grill for 4-5 minutes until the skin is crisp.

Fish grilling sometimes doesn't require flipping since they are fully ready even by grilling just one side.

4. Chicken

There are different ways of preparing a chicken. Below are several ways you can use to prepare your chicken for a tasty meal.

Simmering Method

Simmering is a cooking technique that is similar to boiling. You cook the food by heating liquids you are cooking with. Simmering is a gentle cook, enabling poultry to maintain its structure in ways impossible with other styles of cooking.

First, you need to boil the liquid, be it soup, heavy cream, or water, and then reduce the heat to temperatures below 200 degrees F.

The simmering period differs depending on how big or small your poultry is. Chopped up chicken pieces require a short time to simmer as compared to a whole chicken. Halves boneless chicken breast, require half an hour. Breast halves with bones, winglets, and wings need 35 to 45 minutes to be fully cooked, while drumsticks, thighs, and legs should be simmered for close to one hour. This is due to not just the size of the bird, but the type of meat.

It is vital to note that the internal temperature of a raw chicken should be not less than 165 degrees F. This enables your meat to be fully cooked. Undercooked poultry is dangerous.

Poaching Method

Poaching is a simple and tasty way of cooking your chicken. A poached chicken has low fats, making it juicy and moist.

Poaching chicken can be done the same way we poached our fish above with added cooking times.

Grilling Method

Grilled chicken is a favorite meal for your family. Grilling a chicken varies depending on the chicken part you intend to grill. For example, chicken breasts, boneless and skinless that are 6-8 ounces each take between eight to twelve minutes over direct medium heat equivalent to 350 degrees F. Chicken thigh or bone-in needs to be grilled for slightly half an hour using medium heat indirectly.

5. Pork

The term pork refers to the butchered meat of a pig. Pork can be prepared and eaten in different forms, such as fried, braised, smoked, steamed, grilled, roasted, or boiled. The following are various methods of cooking pork.

Grilling Method

There are two different methods of grilling pork, depending on the size of the cut. For small cuts such as chops, burgers, tenderloin, and kabobs, place the food directly over the heat source.

For significant cuts such as shoulders, ribs, and fresh ham, use indirect heat by placing the meat on the grill rack away from the gas burners or coal.

Always coat the grill bars with fat or lard that has a high smoke point to prevent your meat from sticking to the grill. Small pork cuts require 4 to 5 minutes of cooking on a hot grill, while massive cuts require more extended and longer cooler cooking periods.

Smoking Method

If it's a pork shoulder that you intend to smoke, wrap the piece of meat using a plastic wrap and refrigerate it overnight. Before the cooking time, remove the pork from the fridge one hour before you put it in a smoker. This helps to bring the internal temperature close to room temperature, thus reducing the smoking time.

Smoke the pork until the inner temperature of the thickest portion is 180 degrees F. at that time, the meat will pull much easier and be ready to serve.

Eating enough proteins is the simplest, easiest, and most delicious ways of losing weight and have a good body physique. Ensure your daily meal doesn't miss proteins for a healthy life.

Chapter 5: Meat first choice food

The Carnivore Diet contains only animal products and no other kinds of food. Majorly, people on Carnivore Diet can eat: Fish: Tilapia, lobster, crab, sardines, salmon, herring, mackerel, and so on.

Meat: Pork, organ meats, lamb, beef, chicken, turkey, and so on.

Other animals produce bone broth, bone marrow, lard, eggs and so on.

Low-lactose dairy (a little amount): Butter, rigid cheese, heavy cream, and so on.

Water

In view with some supporters of the Carnivore Diet, pepper, salt as well as seasonings that contain no-carb are permitted.

Also, few people decide to eat milk, soft cheese, and yogurt; however, these kinds of foods are not contained in the carb lists.

Foods to avoid

The kind of foods that do not proceed from animals is exempted from the Carnivore Diet.

Restrained foods include:

- Fruits: berries, bananas, oranges, kiwi, apples.
- Legumes: lentils, beans.
- Alcohol: Liquor, beer.
- Beverages apart from water: tea, fruit juice, coffee, soda.
- Sugars: maple syrup, brown sugar, table sugar.
- Vegetables: Peppers, broccoli, green beans, potatoes, cauliflower.
- Grains: bread, rice, wheat, pasta, quinoa.
- High-lactose dairy: Soft cheese, milk, yogurt, and so on.
- Nuts and seeds: Sunflower seeds, almonds, pumpkin seeds, pistachios.

While people may eat the foods listed above, people who are on the Carnivore Diet are not allowed to eat any of the listed foods.

Chapter 6: Breakfast

Bacon-Wrapped Chicken Liver & Sage

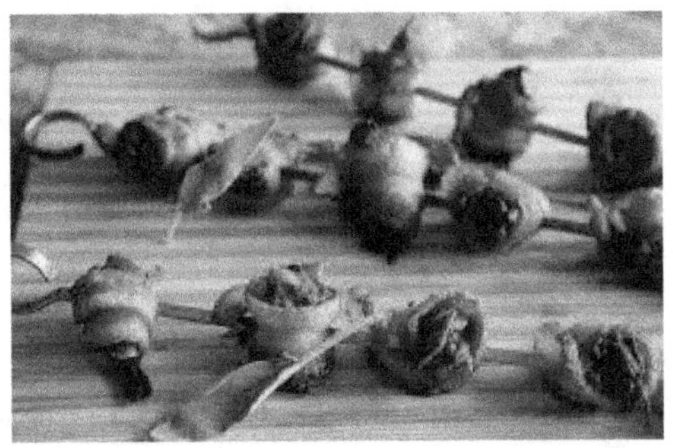

Preparation Time:35 minutes

Serving: 4

Ingredients:

Chicken liver (1 lb.)

Bacon (1 lb.)

Fresh sage (1 pkg.)

Skewers (9-10)

Directions

Heat the oven at 450° Fahrenheit.

Remove the excess veins and fat from the liver, rinse, and pat them dry. Dice each piece into small chunks.

Slice the bacon into halves and add a piece of liver and sage. Stick it on a skewer, leaving space between each one for even cooking.

Bake for 20 to 25 minutes and drain on towels before serving with a garnish of fresh sage.

Nutrition:

Calories: 443 Fat: 34g Carb: 7.2g Protein: 48.1g

Bacon-Wrapped Garlic Chicken Bites

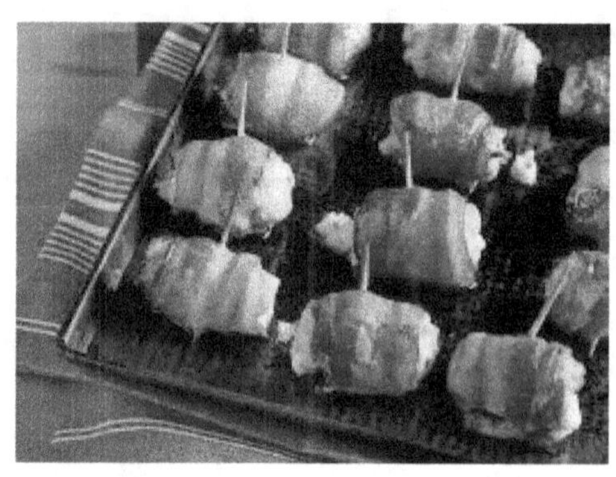

Preparation Time:40 minutes

Servings: 4

Ingredients Needed:

Bite-sized chicken breast (1 large - 22-27 pieces)

Bacon (8-9 thinly sliced strips)

Garlic powder (3 tbsp.) or Crushed garlic (6 cloves)

Directions

Warm the oven to reach 400° Fahrenheit. Prepare a baking pan with a layer of foil.

Slice the bacon into thirds.

Dip the chicken in a dish with the garlic/garlic powder.

Wrap a slice of bacon around each piece of chicken.

Place them onto the tray to bake for 25 to 30 minutes. Flip them over about halfway through the roasting cycle.

Nutrition:

Calories: 400

Fat: 4g

Carb: 2g

Protein: 41g

Bacon-Wrapped Salmon

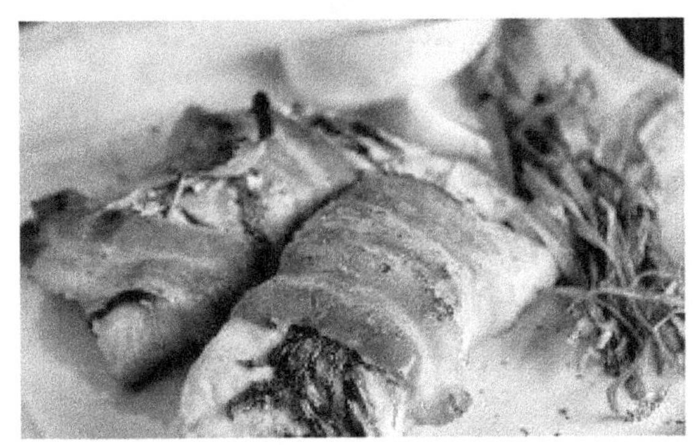

Preparation Time:30 minutes

Serving Yields: 2

Ingredients:

Salmon fillets (2)

Olive oil (1 tbsp.)

Lemon wedges

Bacon slices (4)

Tarragon (2 tbsp.)

Directions

Heat the oven to reach 350° Fahrenheit.

Dry the salmon using a paper towel. Wrap each piece with the bacon.

Arrange the wrapped pieces on a baking tray to roast for 15-20 minutes.

Enjoy it with a sprinkle of chopped tarragon and lemon wedges.

Nutrition:

Calories: 403

Fat: 30g

Carb: 7g

Protein: 48g

Baked Bacon

Preparation Time:15 minutes

Servings: 3

Ingredients:

Sliced bacon (4 slices)

Directions

Warm the oven to reach 350° Fahrenheit.

Arrange the bacon on a baking tray. (You can bake more and use it for snacks.)

Bake them for 15 minutes. Drain on towels, saving the fat in a jar for later (after it's cooled).

Baked Breakfast Casserole Specialty

Preparation Time: 1 hour 15 minutes

Servings: 6-8

Ingredients:

Cooked & crumbled grilled chicken/ground meat (1 lb.)

Eggs (1 dozen)

Optional: Cheese of choice (5-6 oz.)

Directions

Whisk each of the fixings in a mixing container and add to the baking dish.

Set a timer for one hour. Check to see if the center is set. If so, it's ready!

Cool for five or ten minutes and serve.

This one is awesome for freezing.

Nutrition:

Calories: 234 Fat: 4g Carb: 2g Protein: 41g

Carnivore Breakfast Biscuits

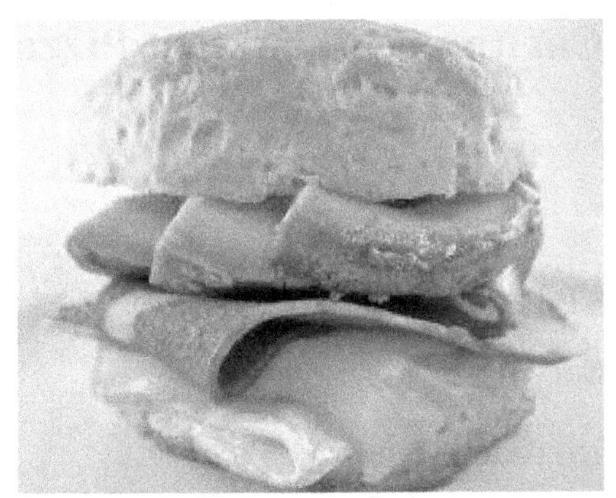

Preparation Time:55-60 minutes

Servings: 10 large biscuits

Ingredients:

Eggs (12)

Optional: Shredded raw cheddar (1 cup)

Your favorite cured meat (varies**)

Unchilled butter (½ stick)

Chicken livers (** 1 in each round)

Directions

Grill the livers in a skillet or grill top to remove its moisture. Set it aside for now.

Warm the oven to reach 350° Fahrenheit.

Grease the cupcake tins with butter and line with the cured meat. Use two if you like a firmer biscuit.

Whisk the eggs until smooth, adding cheese if desired. Fill the cups up to ¾ full.

Arrange the liver in the center of each round and bake for 30 minutes.

** Note: Prepare enough liver and as many slices of your favorite cured meat to place one piece in each cupcake round.

Nutrition:

Calories: 325

Fat: 30g

Carb: 7g

Protein: 41g

Carnivore Breakfast Pizza

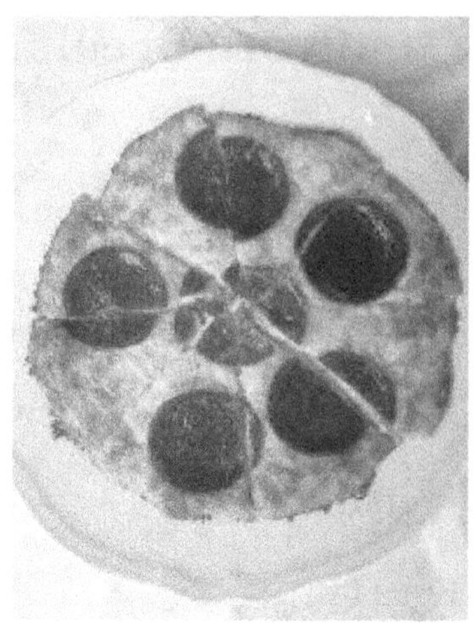

Preparation Time:20 minutes

Servings: 5

Ingredients:

Eggs (8-10)

Bacon (16 oz.)

Pepper and salt (to taste)

Directions

Arrange the package of bacon into a cold skillet.

Set the temperature to medium-high.

As the bacon begins to expel grease, remove the drippings for later. Continue cooking flipping each piece to touch and form the crust of the pizza.

At the point it is about two-thirds done, add the eggs over the top of the bacon.

Lower the temperature setting to medium. When the eggs are set, raise the heat for a crispier texture. Add the pepper and salt to your liking.

Carefully transfer the pizza onto a cutting board and a sheet of parchment paper.

Slice and serve.

Nutrition:

Calories: 245

Fat: 30g

Carb: 7g

Protein: 40g

Chicken Bacon Sausages

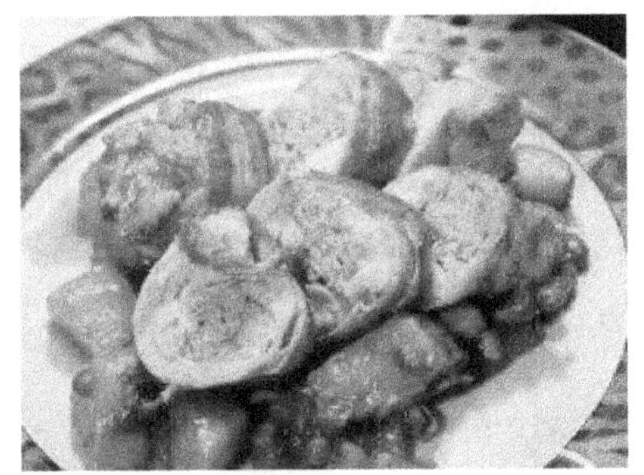

Preparation Time:30 minutes

Servings: 12

Ingredients:

Crumbled bacon bits (2 slices bacon)

Chicken breast (1 lb.)

Egg (1)

Italian seasoning (2 tbsp.)

Pepper & salt (to your liking or .5 tsp. of each)

Garlic powder (2 tsp.)

Onion powder (2 tsp.)

Directions

Program the oven setting to reach 425° Fahrenheit.

Toss all of the fixings into a food processor.

Form 12 (.5-inch) patties and place them onto a foil-lined baking sheet.

Bake until the thermometer reaches 170° Fahrenheit internally or about 20 minutes.

Serve now or freeze them for up to four weeks.

Nutrition:

Calories: 600

Fat: 26g

Carb: 8g

Protein: 78g

Cloud Cake Delight

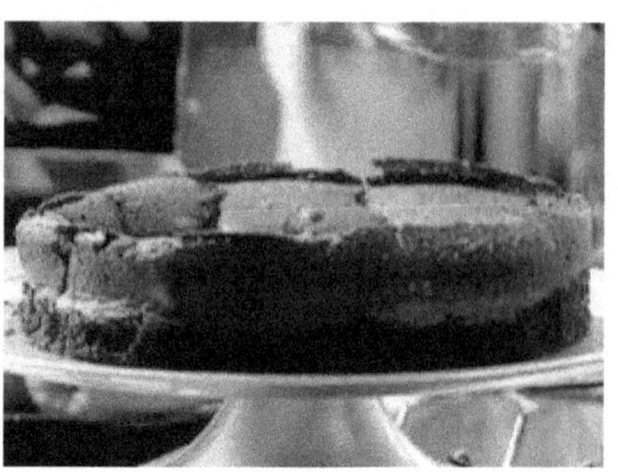

*Preparation Time:*1 hour 10 minutes

Servings: 12

Ingredients:

Eggs (24 whites)

Farmer's cheese (12 oz.)

Shredded raw cheddar (2 cups)

Bacon drippings (2 oz.)

Directions

Whisk the eggs and fold in the cheese.

Grease the baking pan with bacon drippings and add the batter.

Bake them until browned (45 min.).

Nutrition:

Calories: 413

Fat: 3g

Carb: 7g

Protein: 41g

Crispy Ham & Egg Cups

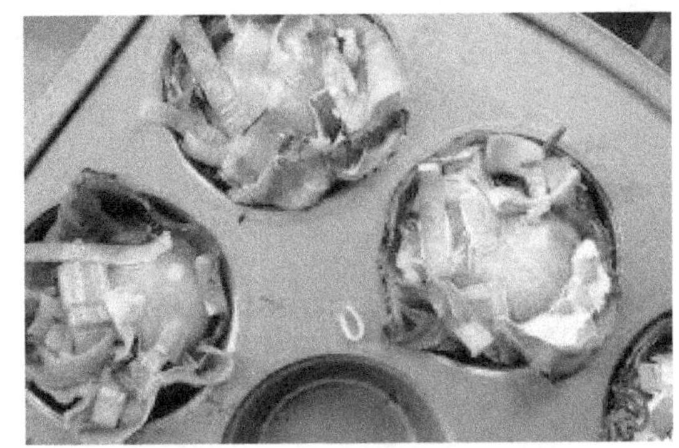

Preparation Time:15 minutes

Servings: 2-4

Ingredients:

Large eggs (4)

Virginia/black forest ham (4 slices)

Pepper and salt (to taste)

Optional: Basil - scallions - fresh parsley

Directions

Set the oven at 400° Fahrenheit. Lightly spritz four muffin cups with cooking oil spray.

Arrange a piece of ham in each slot and add an egg.

Bake them about 13 minutes and remove while the yolks are still runny.

Sprinkle with salt, pepper, and your desired toppings before serving.

Nutrition:

Calories: 356

Fat: 3g

Carb: 12g

Protein: 21g

Easy Egg & Bacon Cups

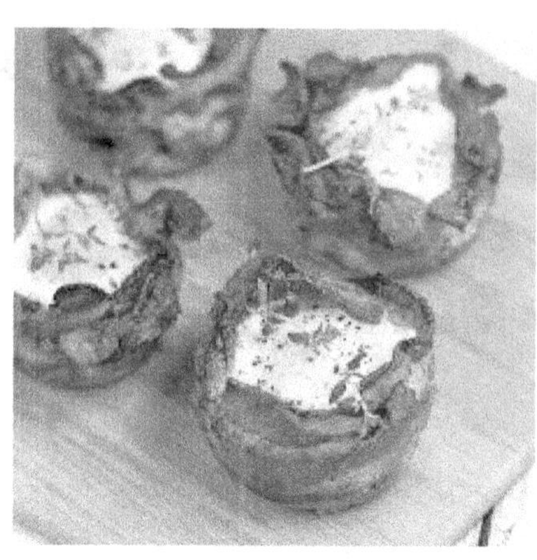

Preparation Time:30 minutes

Servings: 3

Ingredients:

Eggs (3 large)

Bacon slices (3 oz.)

Shredded cheddar cheese (.75 cup)

Pepper and salt (to your liking)

Fresh basil

Directions

Heat the oven to reach 400° Fahrenheit. Spray six muffin cups with cooking oil spray.

Add a piece of bacon, shaping it in each cup with two tablespoons of cheese and one egg. Sprinkle with pepper and salt.

Bake for 12 to 24 minutes until they are set and serve with a garnish of basil.

Nutrition:

Calories: 325

Fat: 4g

Carb: 2g

Protein: 21g

Eggs & Bacon

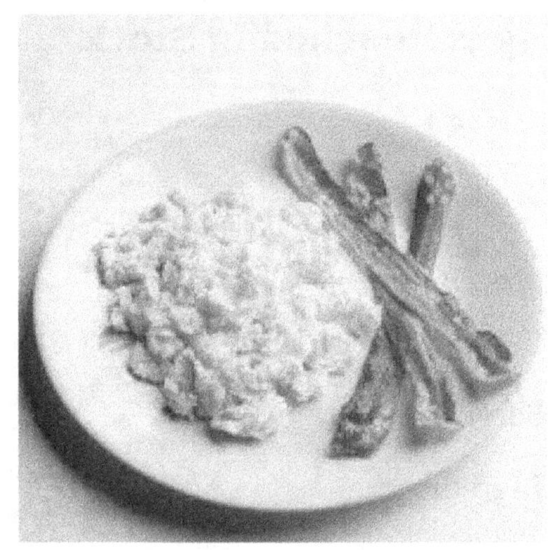

Preparation Time:15 minutes

Servings: 4

Ingredients Needed:

Eggs (8)

Bacon slices (5 oz.)

Fresh parsley

Directions

Fry all of the bacon in one pan and rotate it out if you need more room.

Crack the eggs into the bacon grease, and cook them however you'd like.

○ Over-Easy Eggs: After a few minutes of frying, flip the eggs over and cook again for another few minutes.

○ Sunny-Side Up: Cover the pan with the lid and don't flip them over.

Remove the eggs once they're cooked and season using the parsley before serving.

Nutrition:

Calories: 156

Fat: 30g

Carb: 9g

Protein: 32g

Eggs Poached in Stock

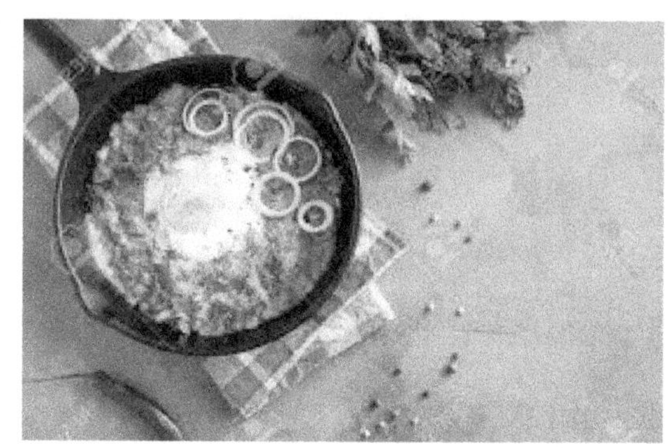

Preparation Time:15 minutes

Servings: 1

Ingredients:

Large eggs (2)

Beef stock (1 cup)

Directions

Add the broth to a large skillet with a lid and wait for it to boil (medium heat).

Crack the eggs in, one at a time, into the broth.

After it begins to simmer, lower the temperature setting to med-low.

Place a lid on the skillet and cook until the white of the egg is solid. Sprinkle it with salt, and remove it from the pan.

Reserve the mixture in the pan as a side with the eggs.

Nutrition:

Calories: 430

Fat: 32g

Carb: 2g

Protein: 41g

Garlic Bacon-Wrapped Chicken Bites

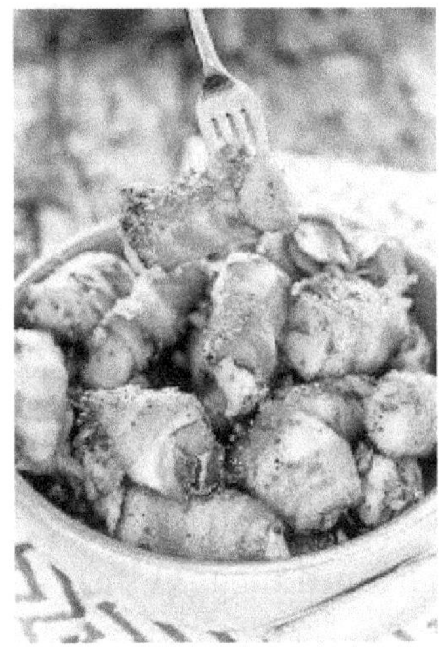

Preparation Time:40 minutes

Servings: 4

Ingredients:

Bacon slices (9)

Large skinless breast of chicken (1)

Garlic powder (3 tbsp.)

Directions

Set the oven to reach 400° Fahrenheit. Prepare a baking sheet with a layer of aluminum foil.

Dice the chicken into small chunks. Slice the bacon into thirds.

Wrap the slices around the chicken and dip them into the garlic powder in a dish.

Arrange them on the baking pan in a single layer.

Bake them until they're crispy or about 25 to 30 minutes.

Nutrition:

Calories: 345

Fat: 35g

Carb: 7g

Protein: 4g

Hidden Treasure Meat Rounds

Preparation Time:2 hours

Servings: 4 rounds

Ingredients:

Ground meat (1 lb.)

Quail eggs (4)

Bacon (4 slices)

Cheese (Optional - 4 small squares - ex. Gouda)

Lard (1 tsp.)

Directions

Prepare the eggs at a boil for about six minutes for hard-boiled.

Portion the ground meat into four mounds. Crack the eggs into the center of the pile and fold it over until the egg is covered.

If you choose, add a slice of cheese on top.

After all four are molded, wrap each one in a strip of bacon.

Use the lard to grease the bottom of the baking pan. Place the rounds into baking pan to bake for 1 hour 45 minutes at 350° Fahrenheit.

Nutrition:

Calories: 167

Fat: 4g

Carb: 5g

Protein: 4.1g

Keto Carnivore Waffle

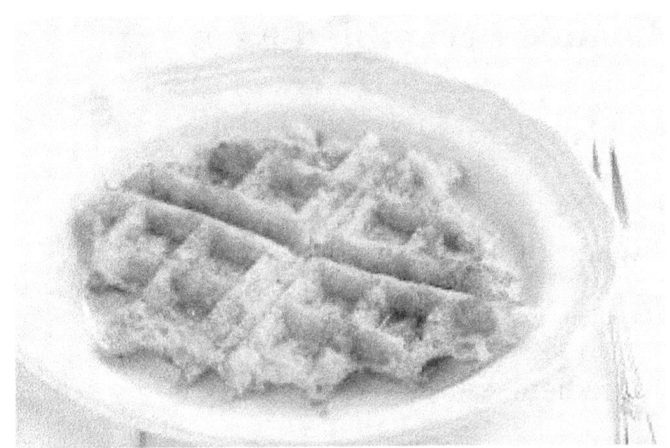

Preparation Time:6 minutes

Servings: 1

Ingredients:

Egg (1)

Ground pork rinds (.5 cup)

Mozzarella cheese (.33 cup)

Salt (1 pinch)

Directions

Warm the waffle maker using the med-high heat setting.

Whisk the fixings in a mixing bowl and pour it into the iron.

Close the waffle iron and cook for three to five minutes, depending on how browned you like them.

Enjoy anytime with just one net carb each!

Nutrition:

Calories: 153

Fat: 4g

Carb: 12g

Protein: 11g

Loaded Scrambled Eggs

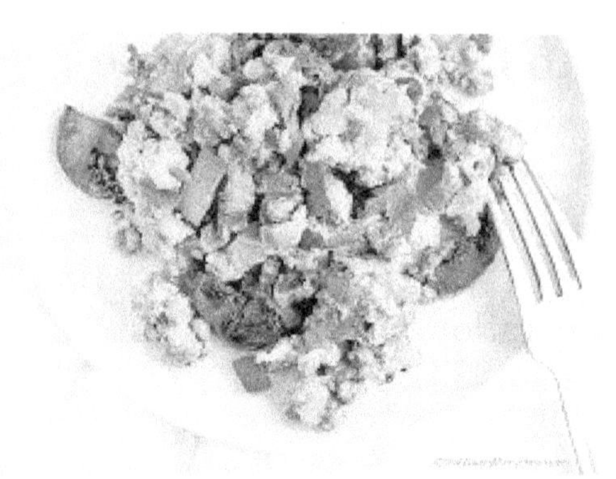

Preparation Time:10-15 minutes

Servings: 4

Ingredients:

Eggs (8)

Sausage (1 lb.)

Sliced bacon (4 chopped)

Pepper and salt (.5 tsp. each)

Tallow/butter (1 tsp.)

Optional: Carnivore-friendly cheese (2 oz.)

Directions

Sauté the sausage, crumbling as it cooks.

Whisk the eggs, salt, and pepper.

Turn the heat down to med-low.

Add the butter to the sausage. Stir in the whisked eggs. Add in the chopped bits of bacon and stir until it's done.

Add cheese when the eggs are plated (if using it).

Nutrition:

Calories: 153

Fat: 4g

Carb: 12g

Protein: 11g

Omelet with Bacon

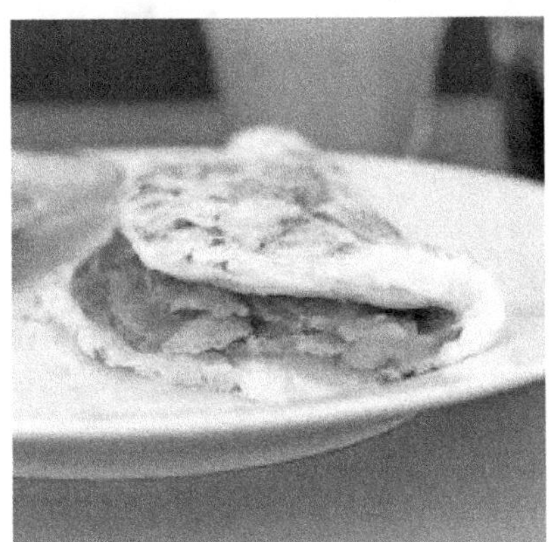

Preparation Time:30 minutes

Servings: 12

Ingredients:

Eggs (4)

Bacon (diced into cubes - 5 oz.)

Butter (3 oz.)

Freshly chopped cloves (1 tbsp.)

Directions

Set the oven at 400° Fahrenheit. Grease a small frying pan with the butter.

Fry the bacon in your remaining butter in a separate pan until crispy. Set it aside. Whisk the eggs and add the bacon to the egg mixture.

Add the chives, salt, and pepper.

Pour the mix into the oven-safe baking dish and bake the omelet for about 20 minutes until it's set.

Enjoy with more bacon if desired.

You can also add grated cheese right out of the oven to melt over the top for extra flavor if desired.

Nutrition:

Calories: 167

Fat: 32g

Carb: 16g

Protein: 21g

Scotch Turkey Eggs

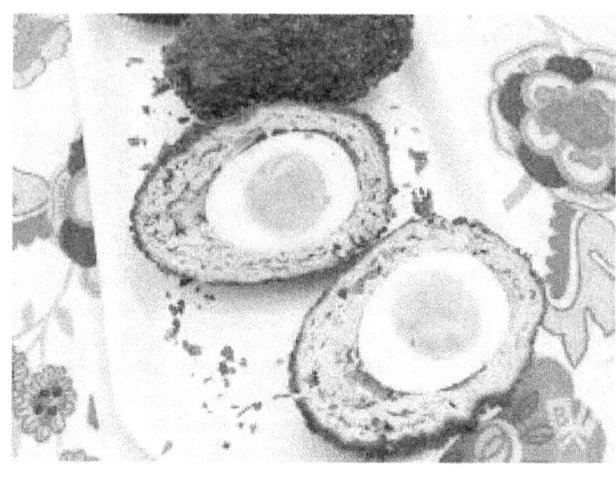

Preparation Time:48-55 minutes

Servings: 6

Ingredients:

Hard-boiled eggs (6)

Ground turkey (1 lb.)

Egg (regular 1)

Garlic powder (2 tsp.)

Cajun seasoning (.5 tbsp.)

Poultry seasoning (1 tsp.)

Grain-Free Breading:

Parmesan cheese (.25 cup)

Salt & black pepper (.5 tsp. each)

Directions

Warm the oven to reach 400° Fahrenheit. Prepare a baking tray with a layer of parchment baking paper.

Mix the turkey, cajun seasoning, garlic powder, and poultry seasoning.

Prepare six patties. Whisk the egg in one dish and add the breading fixings in another. Add the hard-boiled egg onto the patty and roll it into a ball.

Dip it into the egg and then the cheese mixture until covered. Arrange them onto the baking sheet and set a timer for 30 minutes. Broil for two to three minutes to brown them before serving. Enjoy them immediately for the best flavor results.

Nutrition:

Calories: 278 Fat: 3g Carb: 12g Protein: 11g

Seared Bacon Burgers

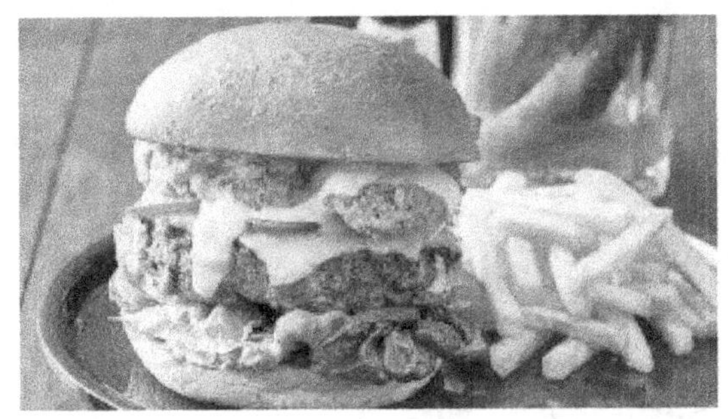

Preparation Time:30 minutes

Servings: 6

Ingredients:

Diced bacon (4 oz.)

Ground beef (1.5 lb.)

Freshly cracked black pepper and salt (.5 tsp.)

Directions

Dice and fry the bacon until it's crunchy.

Save the grease in the skillet.

Prepare the bacon bits and beef with pepper and salt.

Fry the burgers using the high setting for 8 to 10 minutes on each side.

Serve for brunch!

Nutrition:

Calories: 156

Fat: 4g

Carb: 8g

Protein: 4.1g

Skillet Cooked Veal Cutlet For Brunch

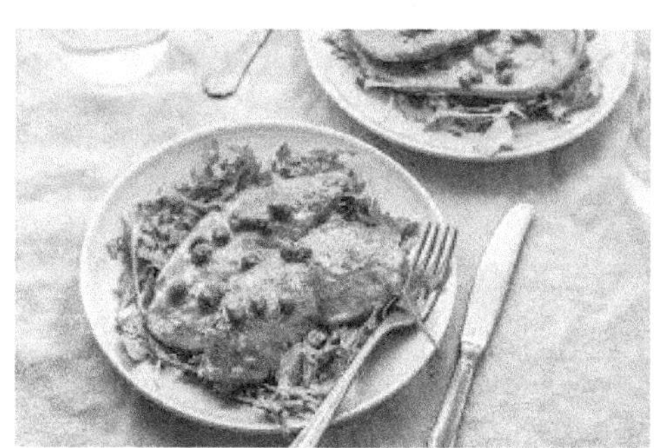

Preparation Time:5-8 minutes

Servings: Varies

Ingredients:

Veal cutlet

Lard or ghee - for cooking

Sea salt (as desired)

Directions

Pound the veal until it's flattened.

Prep a skillet until it's hot with the animal fat of choice.

Dust the veal with salt and add it to the hot skillet and prepare for one minute on each side or as desired.

Nutrition:

Calories: 178

Fat: 3g

Carb: 7g

Protein: 41g

Steak with Egg & Cheese

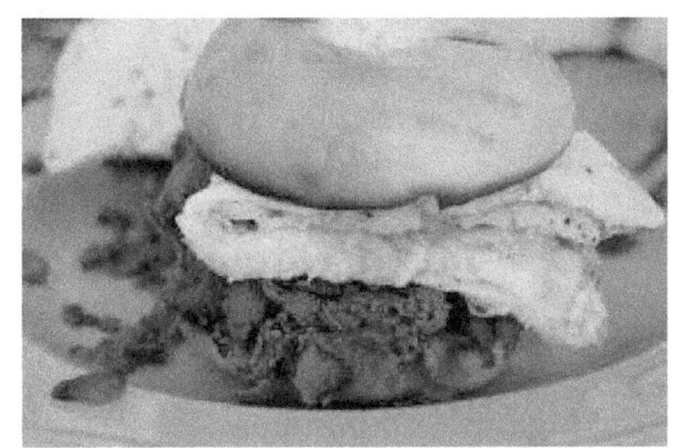

Preparation Time:15-20 minutes

Servings: 1

Ingredients:

Strip steak (8 oz.)

Eggs (1)

Bacon (2 slices if needed)

Directions

Either use reserved bacon grease or prepare a few slices to serve with your meal.

Cook the bacon in a cast-iron skillet using the medium temperature setting.

Leave the bacon slightly soft, and add the steak raising the temperature setting to med-high. Sear the first side of the steak and flip it over.

Adjust the temperature to med-low and continue cooking until it's as you like it or about five minutes.

Fry your egg while the steak rests. Reheat bacon if using and serve.

Nutrition:

Calories: 233

Fat: 4g

Carb: 8g

Protein: 42g

Chapter 7: Seafood

Lemon Baked Salmon

Preparation time: 5 minutes

Cooking time: 20 minutes

Servings: 2

Ingredients:

12 oz filets of salmon

2 lemons, sliced thinly

2 tbsps olive oil

Salt and black pepper, to taste

3 sprigs thyme

Directions:

Preheat the oven to 350° F.

Place half the sliced lemons on the bottom of a baking dish. Place the fillets over the lemons and cover with the remaining lemon slices and thyme.

Drizzle olive oil over the dish and cook for 20 minutes.

Season with salt and pepper.

Nutrition: Carbohydrates: 2 g Fat: 44 g Protein: 42 g Calories: 571

Easy Blackened Shrimp

Preparation time: 10 minutes

Cooking time: 6 minutes

Servings: 2

Ingredients:

½ lb shrimp, peeled and deveined

2 tbsp blackened seasoning

1 tsp olive oil

Juice of 1 lemon

Directions:

Toss all ingredients (except oil) together until shrimp are well coated.

In a non-stick skillet, heat the oil to medium-high heat.

Add shrimp and cook 2-3 minutes per side.

Serve immediately.

Nutrition: Carbohydrates: 5.1 g Fat: 3.9 g Protein: 24.4 g Calories: 152

Grilled Shrimp Easy Seasoning

Preparation time: 5 minutes

Cooking time: 5 minutes

Servings: 4

Ingredients:

For the shrimp seasoning:

1 tsp garlic powder

1 tsp kosher salt

1 tsp Italian seasoning

¼ tsp cayenne pepper

For grilling:

2 tbsps olive oil

1 tbsp lemon juice

1 lb jumbo shrimp, peeled, deveined

Ghee for the grill

Directions:

Preheat the grill pan to high.

In a mixing bowl, stir together the seasoning ingredients.

Drizzle in the lemon juice and olive oil and stir.

Add the shrimp and toss to coat.

Brush the grill pan with ghee.

Grill the shrimp until pink, about 2-3 minutes per side. Serve immediately.

Nutrition: Carbohydrates: 1 g Fat: 3 g Protein: 28 g Calories: 102

The Best Garlic Cilantro Salmon

Preparation time: 10 minutes

Cooking time: 15 minutes

Servings: 4

Ingredients:

1 lb salmon filet

1 tbsp butter

1 lemon

¼ cup fresh cilantro leaves, chopped

4 cloves garlic, minced

½ tsp Kosher salt

½ tsp freshly cracked black pepper

Directions:

Preheat oven to 400° F.

On a foil-lined baking sheet, place salmon skin side down.

Squeeze lemon over the salmon.

Season salmon with cilantro and garlic, pepper and salt.

Slice butter thinly and place pieces evenly over the salmon.

Bake for about 7 minutes, depending on thickness.

Turn the oven to broil and cook 5-7 minutes, until the top is crispy.

Remove salmon from oven and serve immediately.

Nutrition: Carbohydrates: 3.5 g Fat: 4 g Protein: 24.9 g Calories: 140

Aromatic Dover Sole Fillets

Preparation time: 5 minutes

Cooking time: 20 minutes

Servings: 2

Ingredients:

6 Dover Sole fillets

¼ cup virgin olive oil

Zest of 1 lemon

Dash of cardamom powder

1 cup fresh cilantro leaves

Pinch of sea salt

Directions:

Bring the fillets to room temperature.

Set the oven's broiler to high.

Pour half of the oil in an oven tray.

Add half of the cilantro leaves, half of the lemon zest, and the cardamom powder.

Lay the fillets in the mixture and top with the remaining ingredients.

Set under the broiler for about 7-8 minutes or until the fish breaks easily with a fork and it is not transparent.

Serve immediately.

Nutrition: Carbohydrates: 2.9 g Fat: 17.9 g Protein: 18.6 g Calories: 244

Trout with Butter Sauce

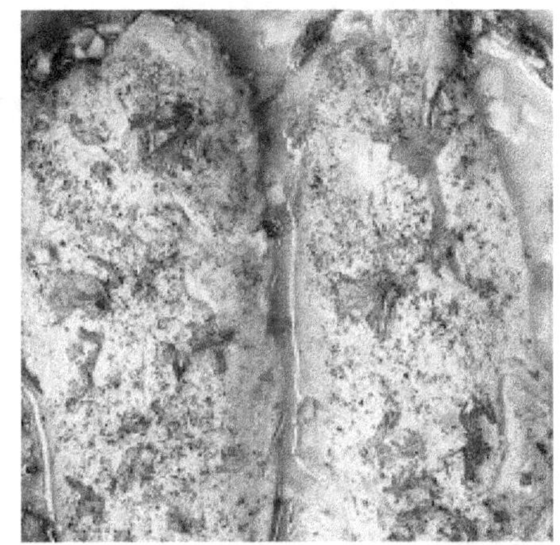

Preparation time: 10 minutes

Cooking time: 10 minutes

Servings: 4

Ingredients

Trout fillets: 4

Salt and ground black pepper to taste

Lemon zest: 3 tsp. [grated].

Fresh chives: 3 Tbsp. [chopped].

Butter: 6 Tbsp.

Olive oil: 2 Tbsp.

Lemon juice: 2 tsp.

Directions:

Season trout with salt, pepper, and drizzle olive oil. Massage into fish.

Heat a kitchen grill over medium heat.

Add fish fillets and cook for 4 minutes. Flip and cook for another 4 minutes.

Heat butter in a pan.

Add lemon juice, lemon zest, chives, salt, and pepper. Mix well.

Divide fish fillets on plates. Drizzle with the butter sauce and serve.

Nutrition:

Calories: 333 Fat: 29.6g Carb: 1g Protein: 16.8g

Roasted Salmon

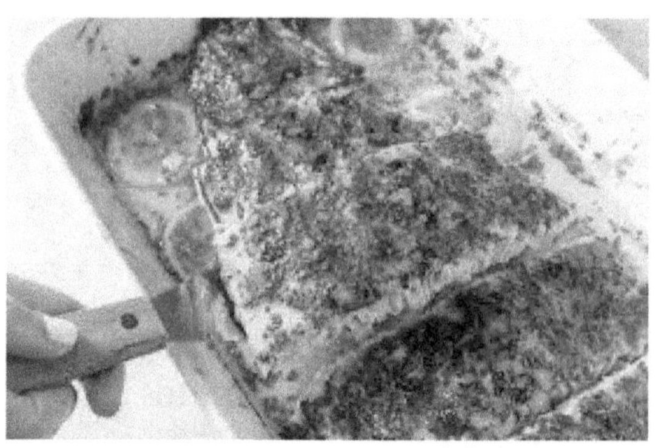

Preparation time: 10 minutes

Cooking time: 12 minutes

Servings: 4

Ingredients

Butter: 2 Tbsp. [softened].

Salmon fillet: 1 ¼ pound

Kimchi: 2 ounces [diced].

Salt and black pepper to taste

Directions:

Mix butter and kimchi in a food processor. Blend well.

Rub salmon with salt, pepper, and kimchi mixture. Place in a baking dish.

Place in an oven at 425F and bake for 15 minutes.

Divide between plates and serve.

Nutrition:

Calories: 467

Fat: 25g

Carb: 1g

Protein: 60g

Salmon Meatballs

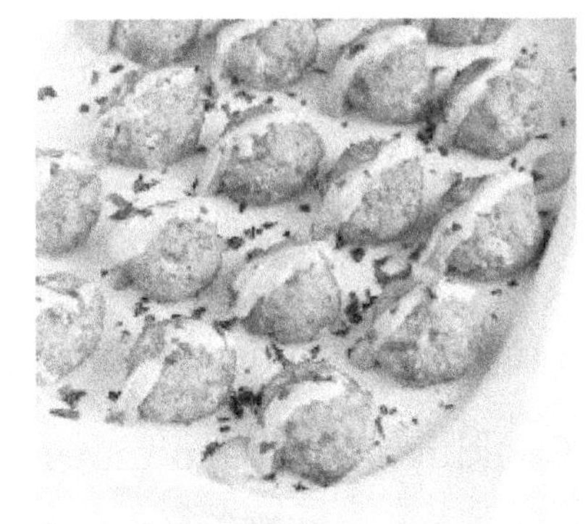

Preparation time: 10 minutes

Cooking time: 30 minutes

Servings: 4

Ingredients:

Butter: 2 Tbsp.

Garlic cloves: 2 [minced].

Onion: 1/3 cup [chopped].

Wild salmon: 1 pound [boneless and minced].

Fresh chives: ¼ cup [chopped]. - Egg: 1

Dijon mustard - 2 Tbsp. - Coconut flour: 1 Tbsp.

Salt and ground black pepper to taste

For the sauce:

Garlic: 4 cloves [minced]. - Butter: 2 Tbsp.

Dijon mustard: 2 Tbsp. - Juice and zest of 1 lemon

Coconut cream: 2 cups - Fresh chives: 2 Tbsp. [chopped].

Directions: Heat 2 tbsp. butter in a pan. Add onion and 2 garlic cloves. Stir-fry for 3 minutes and transfer to a bowl. In another bowl, mix the onion and garlic with salmon, egg, 2 tbsp. mustard, salt, pepper, coconut flour, and chives. Shape meatballs from the salmon mixture and place on a baking sheet. Bake at 350F for 25 minutes. Heat a pan with 2 tbsp. butter over medium heat. Add 4 garlic cloves. Stir-fry for 1 minute. Add chives, lemon juice, lemon zest, 2 tbsp. Dijon mustard, and coconut cream. Cook for 3 minutes. Take salmon meatballs out of the oven; drop them into the Dijon sauce. Toss and cook for 1 minute. Serve.

Nutrition: Calories: 575 Fat: 47.1g Carb: 9g Protein: 31.9g

Salmon with Caper Sauce

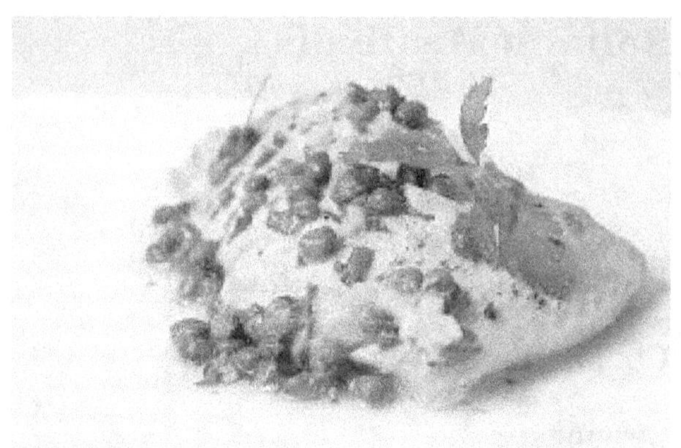

Preparation time: 10 minutes

Cooking time: 20 minutes

Servings: 3

Ingredients

Salmon fillets - 3

Salt and ground black pepper to taste

Olive oil: 1 Tbsp.

Italian seasoning: 1 Tbsp.

Capers: 2 Tbsp.

Lemon juice: 3 Tbsp.

Garlic: 4 cloves [minced].

Butter: 2 Tbsp.

Directions:

Heat olive oil in a pan over medium heat.

Add fish fillets skin side up. Season with salt, pepper, and seasoning.

Cook for 2 minutes, flip and cook for 2 minutes again.

Remove from the heat, cover pan, and set aside for 15 minutes.

Transfer fish to a plate, and leave them aside.

Heat the same pan over medium heat.   Add capers, lemon juice, and garlic. Stir-fry for 2 minutes.

Take the pan off the heat and butter and stir well.   Return fish to the pan and toss to coat with the sauce.   Serve.

Nutrition: Calories: 369 Fat: 24.9g Carb: 2.4g Protein: 35g

Grilled Oysters

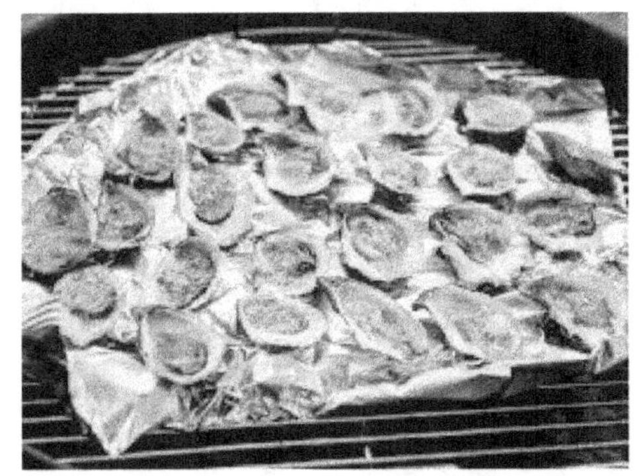

Preparation time: 10 minutes

Cooking time: 10 minutes

Servings: 3

Ingredients

Oysters: 6 [shucked].

Garlic: 3 cloves [peeled and minced].

Lemon: 1 [cut in wedges].

Parsley: 1 Tbsp.

Sweet paprika: 1 pinch

Melted butter: 2 Tbsp.

Directions:

Top each oyster with melted butter, parsley, and paprika.

Place on a preheated grill pan over medium-high heat, and cook for 8 minutes.

Serve them with lemon wedges on the side.

Nutrition:

Calories: 272

Fat: 15.7g

Carb: 3g

Protein: 20.3g

Baked Halibut

Preparation time: 10 minutes

Cooking time: 10 minutes

Servings: 4

Ingredients

Parmesan cheese: ½ cup [grated].

Butter: ¼ cup

Mayonnaise: ¼ cup

Green onions: 2 Tbsp. [chopped].

Garlic: 6 cloves [minced].

Tabasco sauce: 1 dash

Halibut fillets: 4

Salt and ground black pepper to taste

Juice of ½ lemon

Directions:

Season halibut with salt, pepper, and some of the lemon juice.

Place in the baking dish, and cook in the oven at 450F for 6 minutes.

Heat butter in a pan.

Add parmesan cheese, mayonnaise, green onions, Tabasco sauce, garlic, remaining lemon juice, and mix well.

Take fish out of the oven and drizzle cheese sauce all over.

Turn the oven to broil and broil the fish for 3 minutes. Serve.

Nutrition: Calories: 530 Fat: 26.2g Carb: 5.7g Protein: 65.6g

Tuna Cakes

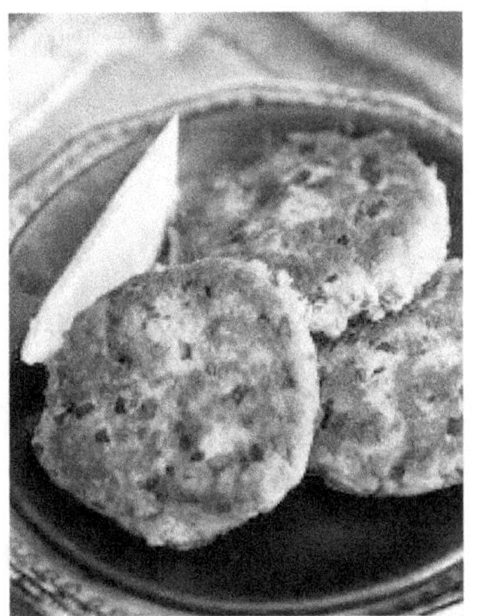

Preparation time: 10 minutes

Cooking time: 10 minutes

Servings: 12

Ingredients

Canned tuna: 15 ounces [drained well and flaked].

Eggs: 3

Dried dill: ½ tsp.

Dried parsley: 1 tsp.

Onion chopped: ½ cup

Garlic powder: 1 tsp.

Salt and ground black pepper to taste

Oil for frying

Directions:

In a bowl, mix the tuna well with salt, pepper, dill, parsley, onion, garlic powder, eggs.

Shape tuna cakes and place on a plate.

Heat cooking oil in a pan.

Add tuna cakes and cook for 5 minutes on each side.

Serve.

Nutrition: Calories: 84 Fat: 4g Carb: 1g Protein: 10.8g

Pan-Roasted Cod

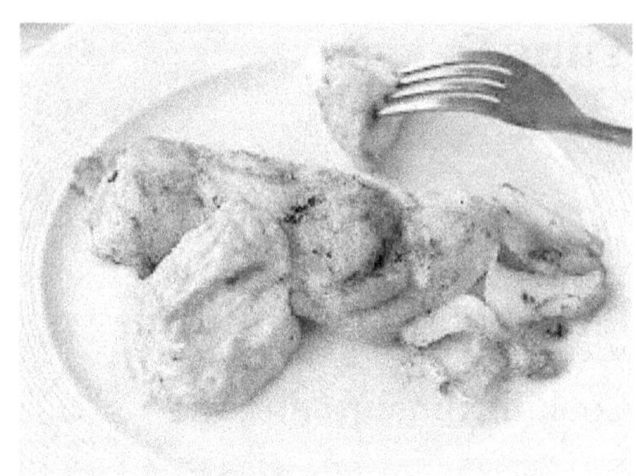

Preparation time: 10 minutes

Cooking time: 20 minutes

Servings: 4

Ingredients

Cod: 1 pound [cut into medium-sized pieces].

Salt and ground black pepper to taste

Green onion: 2 [chopped].

Garlic: 3 cloves [minced].

Liquid anions: 3 Tbsp.

Fish stock: 1 cup

Balsamic vinegar: 1 Tbsp.

Fresh ginger: 1 Tbsp. [grated].

Red chili flakes: ½ tsp.

Directions:

Brown the fish pieces in a pan on all sides.

Add ginger, chili pepper, vinegar, fish stock, liquid aminos, salt, pepper, green onions, and garlic.

Stir and cover. Lower the heat and cook for 20 minutes.

Divide between plates and serve.

Nutrition: Calories: 131 Fat: 1g Carb: 2.2g Protein: 26.9g

Sea Bass with Capers

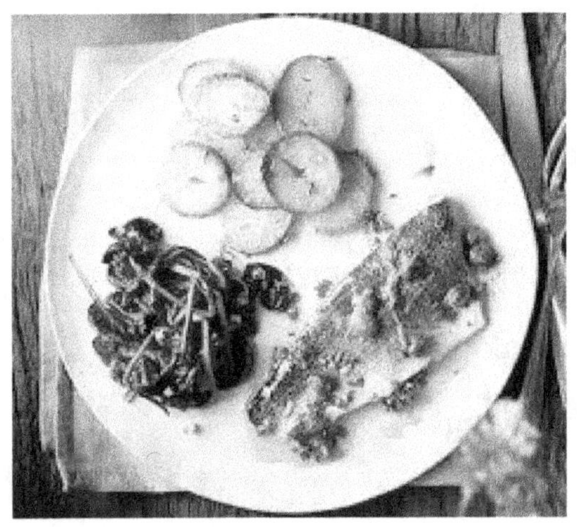

Preparation time: 10 minutes

Cooking time: 15 minutes

Servings: 4

Ingredients

Lemon: 1 sliced

Sea bass fillet: 1 pound

Capers: 2 Tbsp.

Fresh dill: 2 Tbsp.

Salt and ground black pepper to taste

Directions:

Place seas bass fillet into a baking dish.

Season with salt, and pepper.

Add capers, dill, and lemon slices on top.

Place in the oven at 350F and bake for 15 minutes.

Serve.

Nutrition:

Calories: 150

Fat: 3.1g

Carb: 2.4g

Protein: 27.4g

Fish Curry

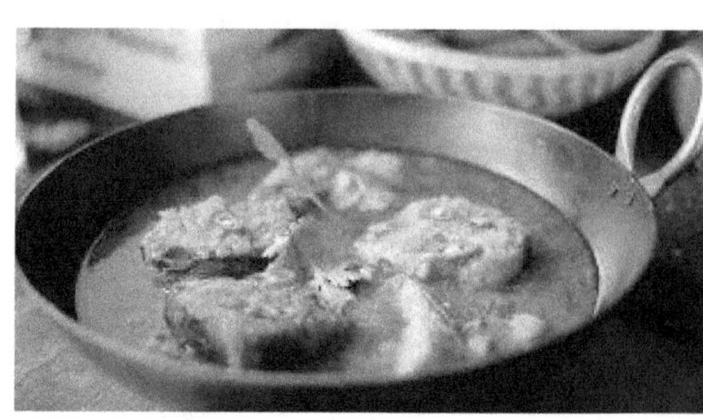

Preparation time: 10 minutes

Cooking time: 25 minutes

Servings: 4

Ingredients

Whitefish fillets: 4

Mustard seeds: ½ tsp.

Salt and black pepper to taste

Green chilies: 2 [chopped].

Fresh ginger: 1 tsp. [grated].

Curry powder: 1 tsp.

Cumin: ¼ tsp. - Coconut oil: 4 Tbsp.

Onion: 1 [chopped].

Turmeric root: 1 inch [grated].

Fresh cilantro: ¼ cup - Coconut cream: 1 ½ cups

Garlic: 3 cloves [minced].

Directions:

Heat half of the coconut oil in a saucepan. Add mustard seeds, and cook for 2 minutes. Add garlic, onion, and ginger and stir-fry for 5 minutes. Add cumin, chilies, curry powder, and turmeric. Cook for 5 minutes. Add salt, pepper, and coconut milk and stir. Bring to a boil and cook for 15 minutes. Heat the remaining oil in a pan over medium heat. Add fish, stir and cook for 3 minutes. Add to curry sauce, stir, and cook for 5 minutes. Add cilantro, stir and serve.

Nutrition: Calories: 541 Fat: 38g Carb:8.8 g Protein: 60.9g

Sautéed Lemon Shrimp

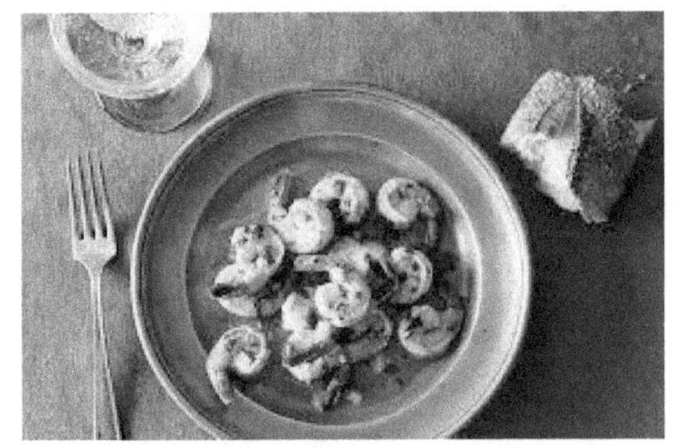

Preparation time: 10 minutes

Cooking time: 10 minutes

Servings: 4

Ingredients

Olive oil: 2 Tbsp.

Butter: 1 Tbsp.

Shrimp: 1 pound [peeled and deveined].

Lemon juice: 2 Tbsp.

Garlic: 2 Tbsp. [minced].

Lemon zest: 1 Tbsp.

Salt and ground black pepper to taste

Directions:

Heat oil and butter in a pan.

Add shrimp and cook for 2 minutes.

Add garlic, stir-fry for 4 minutes.

Add salt, pepper, lemon juice, and lemon zest. Stir and take off the heat.

Serve.

Nutrition:

Calories: 220

Fat: 11.8g

Carb: 1.7g

Protein: 25.9g

Coconut Shrimp

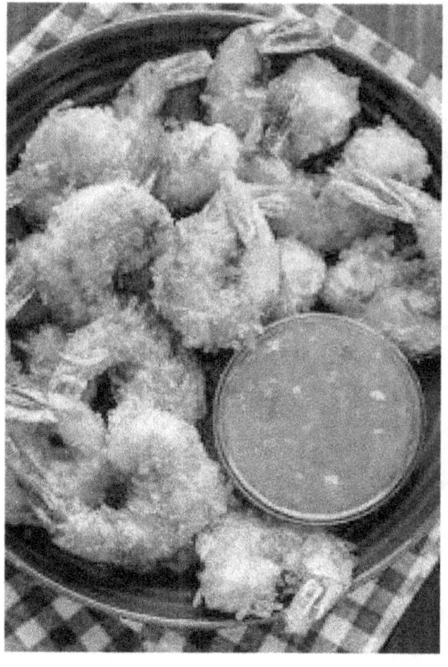

Preparation time: 10 minutes

Cooking time: 13 minutes

Servings: 4

Ingredients

Shrimp: 1 pound [peeled and deveined].

Salt and ground black pepper to taste

Cherry tomatoes: 4 [chopped].

Red bell pepper: 1 [seeded and sliced].

Olive oil: 1 Tbsp.

Fresh cilantro: ½ cup [chopped].

Garlic: 1 Tbsp. [minced].

Green onion: ½ cup [chopped].

Red pepper flakes: ½ tsp.

Coconut milk: 10 ounces

Lime juice: 2 Tbsp.

Directions:

Heat olive oil in a pan.

Add pepper and cook for 3 minutes.

Add pepper flakes, green onions, garlic, and cilantro. Cook for 1 minute.

Add coconut milk, and tomatoes, stir and simmer for 5 minutes.   Add lime juice and shrimp, stir and cook for 3 minutes.   Season with salt and pepper, stir and serve.

Nutrition: Calories: 368 Fat: 22.7g Carb: 4.7g Protein: 29.3g

Bacon-Wrapped Salmon

Preparation time: 10 minutes

Cooking time: 20 minutes

Servings: 2

Nutrition: Carbohydrates: 7.1 g Fat −42 g Protein: 53.3 g Calories: 612

Ingredients:

2 salmon fillets

1 tbsp olive oil

4 slices bacon

Lemon wedges

2 tbsp tarragon

Directions:

Preheat the oven to 350°F.

Pat the filets dry.

Wrap bacon around the salmon filets.

Place filets on a roasting tray, and drizzle with the olive oil.

Bake for 15-20 minutes.

Garnish with lemon wedges and chopped tarragon.

Japanese Fish Bone Broth

Preparation time: 5 minutes

Cooking time: 4 hours

Servings: 6-8

Nutrition: Carbohydrates: 0 g Fat: 2 g Protein: 5 g Calories: 40

Ingredients:

Fish head and carcass

4 slices ginger

1 tbsp lemon juice

½ leek, sliced

Sea salt, to taste

Water

Directions:

Place the fish head and carcass into a large pot with cold water.

Bring to a boil and pour out the water.

Refill the pot with fresh water and add in the leek, sea salt, ginger, and lemon juice.

Simmer, covered, about 4 hours.

Garlic Ghee Pan-Fried Cod

Preparation time: 5 minutes

Cooking time: 10 minutes

Servings: 4

Nutrition: Carbohydrates: 1 g Fat: 7 g Protein: 21 g Calories: 160

Ingredients:

1¼ lb cod fillets

3 tbsps ghee

6 cloves of garlic, minced

1 tbsp garlic powder

A pinch salt

Directions:

In a frying pan on medium-high heat, melt the ghee.

Add half the minced garlic.

Place the cod fillets in the pan and sprinkle with garlic powder and salt.

Cook until fish is a solid white color, about 4-5 minutes. Then flip the fillets and add the remaining minced garlic. Cook until the whole fillets turn a solid white color, about 4-5 minutes.

Serve with the ghee and garlic from the pan.

Steam Your Own Lobster

Preparation time: 10 minutes

Cooking time: 10 minutes

Servings: 4

Ingredients:

4 lobster tails

1 sprig parsley

Directions:

If the lobster tails are frozen, defrost them.

Before cooking, make a long slit in the underbelly of the lobster.

Fill a pot halfway with water. Place a steamer basket inside.

Once the water is boiling, place the lobster tails onto the steamer attachment.

Let boil for for 8-9 minutes for fresh lobster and 10 minutes for defrosted lobster.

Garnish with parsley.

Recipe Notes: If using fresh lobster, steam it for 8-9 minutes.

Nutrition: Carbohydrates: 0 g Fat: 0 g Protein: 24 g Calories: 100

Thyme Roasted Salmon

Preparation time: 10 minutes

Cooking time: 20 minutes

Servings: 4

Ingredients:

1 lb fresh salmon, skinless

2 tsp olive oil

¼ tsp kosher salt

1 tbsp ghee

½ tsp dried thyme

Lemon wedges

Directions:

Preheat oven to 400° F.

Cut salmon into four equal-sized pieces.

Line a sheet pan with parchment paper and place salmon on it.

Brush with olive oil and season with salt.

Roast for 10 minutes.

In a small bowl, mix dried thyme and ghee. Set aside.

After 10 minutes of cooking, brush salmon with thyme-ghee mixture.

Roast for 5-8 minutes more, or until salmon is just cooked through.

Before serving, allow to rest for 10 minutes.

Nutrition: Carbohydrates: 0 g Fat: 9 g Protein: 25 g Calories: 186

Pan-Fried Tilapia

Preparation time: 10 minutes

Cooking time: 10 minutes

Servings: 4

Ingredients:

2 tilapia filets

Salt, to taste

2 tbsps coconut oil

Directions:

Add coconut oil to a frying pan on medium heat.

Salt the tilapia fillets.

Place the fillets in the frying pan and cook until fish is a solid white color, about 4-5 minutes. Then flip the fillets and cook until the whole fillets turn a solid white color, about 4-5 minutes.

Serve immediately.

Nutrition: Carbohydrates: 0.7 g Fat: 1 g Protein: 21 g Calories: 91

Calamari Rings

Preparation time: 5 minutes

Cooking time: 2 minutes

Servings: 4

Ingredients:

4 calamari squid tubes

1 tbsp ghee

2 tbsp almond flour

Zest and juice of 1 lemon

Salt and pepper, to taste

Directions:

Mix the almond flour, lemon zest, salt, and pepper.

Slice the squid tubes into ½-inch slices.

Roll the calamari rings in the almond mix.

Heat ghee in a frying pan and fry rings on low heat for 1 minute each side until cooked and golden.

Drizzle with lemon juice.

Nutrition: Carbohydrates: 5.9 g Fat: 8.2 g Protein: 16.3 g Calories: 159

Chapter 8: Appetizers salads and sides

Bacon Wrapped Lobster Chunks and Egg Dip

Preparation time: 15 minutes

Cooking time: 15 minutes

Servings: 3-4

Ingredients:

1 lb lobster tail - 9 strips of bacon

Salt and pepper to taste

Dipping Sauce

1 egg - ½ tsp salt

Pinch of pepper - Butter, as may be needed

Directions: Remove the lobster tail shell and fry the meat on a pan for 5 minutes each side using 2 tablespoons of butter. Continue bathing the lobster meat in butter until all sides are soft and sprinkle with salt. Remove from the pan and slice along the natural tail grooves into 1½ inch chunks. Slice your bacon into strips. Wrap the lobster chunks with your bacon strips and secure the roll with a toothpick. Separately arrange your rolls on a buttered baking sheet ensuring they don't run into each other. Place them in an oven and broil using the second highest level. Continue to broil for 10 minutes, flipping each roll over in the middle. Dipping In a blender, add the egg, teaspoon of butter, salt, and pepper. Blend until the mixture turns light in color. By now, the rolls are crisp and ready. Remove and place them on a serving plate. Enjoy your dip.

Calories per serving: 364 Kcal

Nutrition: Calories: 443 Fat: 34g Carb: 7.2g Protein: 48.1g

Beef Jerky

Cooking time: 10 minutes

Preparation time: 12 hours

Servings: 12

Ingredients

2 pounds of beef brisket or steak or sirloin

 Brine:

½ tsp salt

1/3 tsp pepper black, ground

1 tsp onion powder

1/3 tsp garlic powder

2 tbsp liquid smoke

½ cup soy sauce

Directions:

Cut beef across grain into 12 slices

Mix the ingredients for the brine and pour over beef slices.

Put them in the refrigerator for the night

After the meat is marinated well, place the slices on the bacon rack in a microwave oven.

Put the paper napkin on the slices and cook for 2 min on high power.

Then turn the slices and cook for another 2 min.

Let them stay in the oven for 5 min before eating.

Enjoy

Tip: the cooking time depends on the beef slices thickness Calories per serving: 150 Kcal

Nutrition: Calories: 443 Fat: 34g Carb: 7.2g Protein: 48.1g

Cocktail Meatballs

Cooking time: 20 minutes

Preparation time: 15 minutes

Servings: 8

Ingredients

1 1/3 pound ground turkey

1 tsp salt

½ tsp black pepper, ground

1/3 cup chicken broth

1 egg

115 g cream cheese

3 tbsp butter

Directions:

Mix all the ingredients together.

Form the balls from the mixture.

Heat up the butter over medium-high heat and brown balls from all sides until the meat is not pink.

Calories per serving: 264 Kcal

Nutrition:

Calories: 233

Fat: 4g

Carb: 7g

Protein: 31g

Sea Scallops

Cooking time: 8 minutes

Preparation time: 5 minutes

Servings: 2

Ingredients

10 sea scallops

3 tbsp butter

Salt and pepper to taste

 Directions:

Season scallops with salt and pepper.

Heat butter over medium-high heat in a skillet.

Place there the scallops and fry from both sides until they are ready.

Use the butter from the skillet as a sauce.

Serve

Calories per serving: 269 Kcal

Nutrition:

Calories: 330

Fat: 30g

Carb: 9g

Protein: 40g

Lamb Kebab

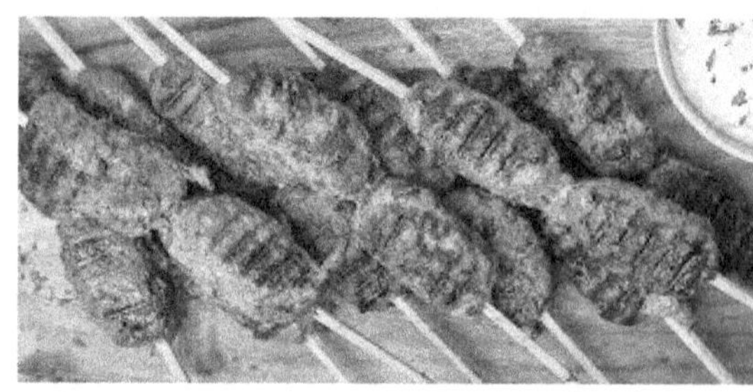

Cooking time: 10 minutes

Preparation time: 10 minutes

Servings: 4

Ingredients

2 pounds diced lamb leg steaks

½ tsp salt

½ tsp black pepper ground

1 tbsp oregano dried

1 clove garlic, grated

2 tbsp fresh lemon juice

 Directions:

Mix all dry ingredients and add lamb slices to marinade.

Put the lamb into the fridge for 1.5-2 hours.

Take out of the fridge and let it stay a few minutes to become a room temperature.

Put the lambs onto the skewers (8 pieces)

Prepare your grill and cook for 4 min each side.

Sprinkle with lemon juice.

Serve and enjoy!

Calories per serving: 455 Kcal

Nutrition:

Calories: 343 Fat: 4g Carb: 12g Protein: 4.1g

Grilled Beef Patties

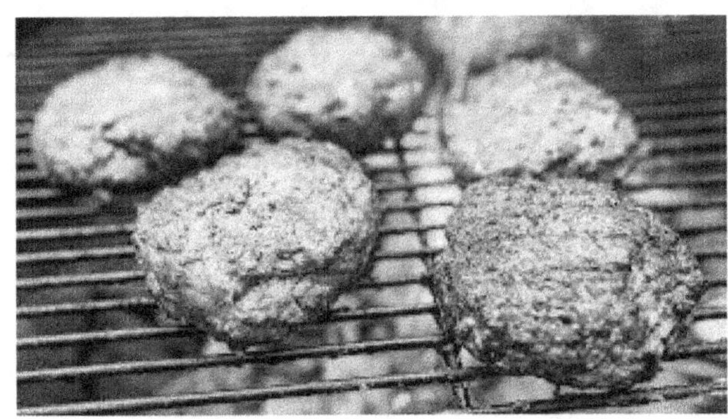

Preparation time: 30 minutes

Cooking time: 20 minutes

Servings: 8

Ingredients

2 pounds ground beef

1 tablespoon lard melted

1/2 teaspoon salt

8 slices Gruyere or aged Swiss cheese

Fried Eggs:

2 tablespoons butter

8 large Free Range Eggs

 Directions:

Beef

Combine the ground beef, melted lard, salt, and mix lightly.

Shape the mixture into eight patties and grill for 7 minutes on each side covered over medium heat until temperatures read 160°F. Eggs. Using two large skillets melt 1 tablespoon of butter on each over medium heat on a grill. Break 4 eggs into a saucer and gently slide them into pans and reduce the heat to low. Place the eggs with the sunny-side facing up and cover the pan. Cook for 4 minutes until the yolks thicken but not hard. If you prefer basted eggs, smear additional butter over the eggs as you continue cooking. Flip the eggs until all the sides are properly cooked. Place the Gruyere slices on top of each egg until they start melting. Serve while hot.

Calories per serving: 595 Kcal

Nutrition: Calories: 167 Fat: 30g   Carb: 7g Protein: 40g

Chorizo Sausage and Bacon Bake

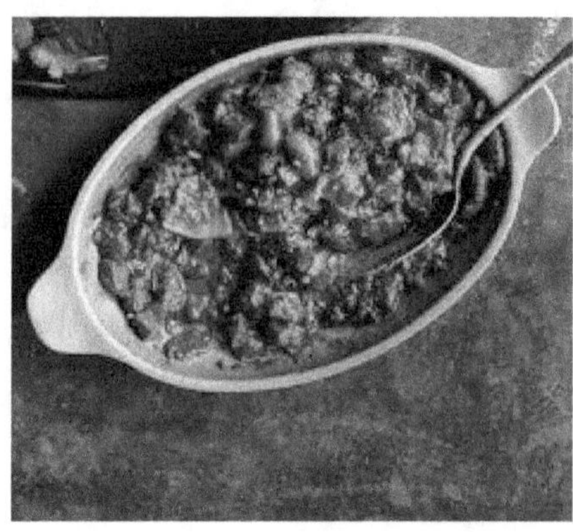

Preparation time: 10 minutes

Cooking time: 13 minutes

Servings: 2

Ingredients

2 tablespoon tallow or lard

1 teaspoon butter

4 ounces chorizo sausage

2 large eggs

Salt to taste

3 slices of cooked and thick-cut bacon

 Directions:

Preheat your oven to 350°F

Using the butter, lightly grease two ramekins.

Heat the tallow or lard over medium-high heat for 3 minutes.

Chop your chorizo sausage and divide equal amounts into each ramekin.

Gently crack an egg into each ramekin.

Season with salt.

Bake for 13 minutes.

Throw bacon on top and serve.

Calories per serving: 450 Kcal

Nutrition: Calories: 421 Fat: 4g Carb: 9g Protein: 8g

Bacon-Wrapped Meatloaf

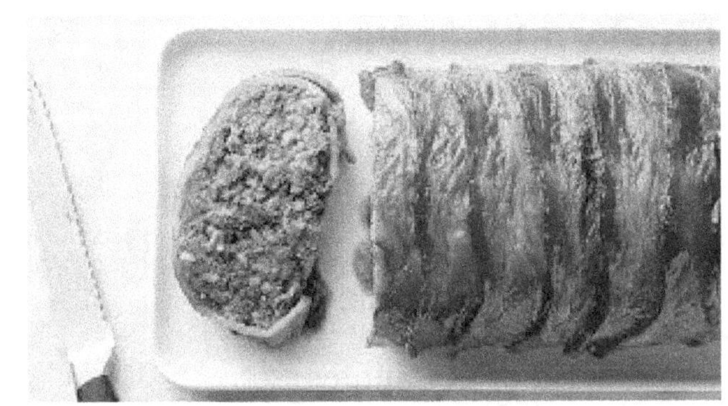

Preparation time: 5 minutes

Cooking time: 25 minutes

Servings: 2 loaves for 4

 Ingredients

1/2 pound ground beef

1/2 pound ground pork

3 tablespoons butter

1 egg

1 cup parmesan cheese

Strips of bacon

Lard

Kosher salt

Directions:

Preheat your oven to 350°F.

In a large bowl, mix the ground pork, beef, egg, parmesan cheese, and salt to taste ensuring the mixture holds together.

Form two small logs using the meat mixture and individually tie them with bacon strips starting from the top. In the meantime, add the butter in a sauté pan and heat on high. Place the bacon meatloaf with the seam side facing downwards to prevent spillage. Flip to cook on both sides until brown.   Transfer the meatloaves into a hot oven and cook for 15 minutes. When the 15 minutes elapses, allow them to rest, slice, and serve.

Calories per serving: 334 kcal

Nutrition: Calories: 443 Fat: 34g Carb: 7.2g Protein: 48.1g ì

Chicken Liver Pate

Preparation time: 5 minute

Cooking time: 25 minutes

Servings: 2 loaves for 4

 Ingredients

0.5 pound chicken liver (1 cup)

½ cup butter

2 tbsp double cream

Salt and pepper to taste

Rosemary sprig

Directions:

Melt 1 tbsp of butter in a frying pan and put the chopped liver. Cook for 8 min.

Place the liver into a food processor and add there butter from the pan and cheese.

Melt two more tbsp. of butter with rosemary, thyme, salt and pepper and add this mixture to the liver.

Blend the liver until it is smooth.

Place the pate into ramekins.

Melt the rest of the butter and cover the pate with it.

Put the rosemary leaves on the top.

Cool in the fridge and serve.

Calories per serving: 365 Kcal

Nutrition: Calories: 123 Fat: 4g Carb: 2g Protein: 41g

Chapter 9: Beef, lamb, pork Recipes

Mongolian Beef Noodles

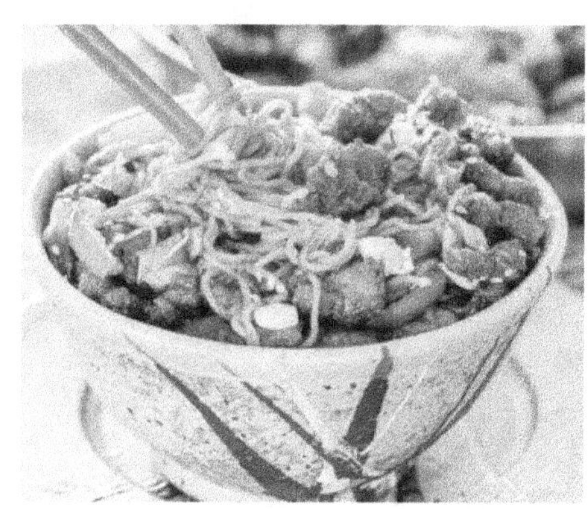

Servings: 4-5

Preparation time: 35 minutes

Ingredients:

1 tbsp. of oil, canola

1 pound of thinly sliced flank steak

1/4 cup of arrow root

1/2 cup of soy sauce, low sodium - 1/2 cup of water, filtered

1/4 cup of honey, pure - 2 minced cloves of garlic

2 tsp. of minced ginger, fresh - 1 tsp. of sriracha sauce

1 pound of noodles, brown rice - 1/2 cup of cucumbers, julienned

1/2 cup of carrots, julienned - 1/4 cup of of sliced green onions

Directions: Add arrow root and flank steak to large size zipper top plastic bag. Toss and coat steak with the arrow root. Don't overmix them. Set the bag aside. Add water, soy sauce, sriracha, ginger, garlic cloves and honey to sauce pan. Bring to boil. Reduce heat and simmer for 8-12 minutes. Heat large sized skillet on med high. Add canola oil. Add flank steak. Sauté for three to four minutes, till steak has browned slightly. Add sriracha sauce from step 2. Cover. Cook for two to three minutes and remove skillet from heat. Bring large pot of filtered water to boil. Add noodles. Then cook for four to six minutes, till barely tender. Remove the noodles and run them under cold tap water. Serve the sauce-covered beef on noodles with green onions, carrots and cucumbers.

Nutrition: Calories: 443 Fat: 34g Carb: 7.2g Protein: 48.1g

Slow Cooker Braised Beef

Servings: 4

Preparation time: 10 minutes + 8 hours slow cooker time

Ingredients:

1 cup of chopped onions, refrigerated

Nonstick spray

1 lb. of trimmed top round steak, boneless

1 x 14 1/2 oz. can of tomatoes, diced, with oregano

and basil, including juice

1/2 cup of beer, light

2 tbsp. of molasses, pure

1/4 tsp. of salt, kosher

Directions:

Spray a medium slow cooker with nonstick spray. Place onions in it.

Heat large skillet on medhigh. Coat with nonstick spray. Add the steak and cook for three minutes per side, till browned. Place steak on top of onions in the slow cooker. Pour the beer and tomatoes over the steak.

Cover slow cooker. Cook on the LOW setting for eight hours. Steak should be very tender.

Next, shred the steak while in the slow cooker. Add and stir salt and molasses. Allow the steak to set for 8-10 minutes. Serve.

Nutrition: Calories: 178 Fat: 3g Carb: 2g Protein: 11g

Lamb Chops Pesto

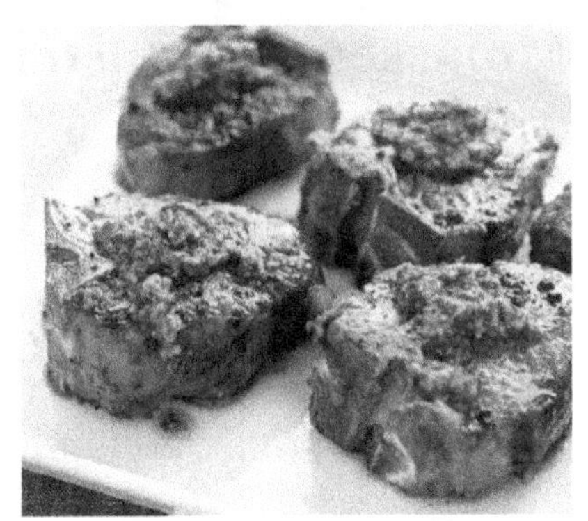

Servings: 4

Preparation time: 20 minutes

8 x 4-oz. trimmed lamb loin chops, lean

1/2 tsp. of salt, kosher

1/2 tsp. of pepper, black, ground

Nonstick spray

1 lemon, fresh

1 tbsp. of toasted pine nuts

2 cloves of garlic

4 cups of arugula leaves, baby

2 tsp. of oil, olive

2 tbsp. of water filtered

Directions:

Preheat the broiler.

Evenly sprinkle the lamb with 1/4 tsp. of kosher salt 1/4 tsp. of ground pepper. Coat a broiler pan with nonstick spray and arrange the lamb in one layer on it. Broil for five to six minutes per side till done as you desire.

As lamb is broiling, grate 1 tsp. of lemon rind. Squeeze the juice from the lemon till you have 2 tsp.

Place garlic and pine nuts in food processor and process till minced. Add the lemon juice, lemon rind, 2 tbsp. of water, oil, arugula, and remainder of kosher salt ground pepper. Process till smooth. Serve the pesto with the lamb.

Nutrition: Calories: 234 Fat: 30g Carb: 7g Protein: 31g

Molasses and Mustard Flank Steak

Servings: 4

Preparation time: 20 minutes + 1/2-hour marinating time

Ingredients:

1/3 cup of vinegar, balsamic

1/4 cup of beef broth, reduced sodium, fat-free

2 tbsp. of molasses, organic

2 tbsp. of Dijon mustard, whole-grain

1/4 tsp. of salt, kosher

1/4 tsp. of pepper, black, ground

1 x 1-lb. of trimmed flank steak

Nonstick spray

Optional: green onions, chopped

Directions:

Combine the first seven ingredients in large zipper top bag and seal. Place in fridge for 1/2 hour to marinate.Preheat the broiler. Next, remove the steak from zipper top bag. Reserve the marinade. Coat a broiler pan with nonstick spray and place steak on it. Broil for five minutes per side, or till it's done to your preferred level. Remove the steak from the oven and cover loosely using foil. Place the reserved marinade in nonstick skillet. Bring to boil and cook till it reduces to about 1/3 of a cup. Stir it occasionally.

Cut the steak across the grain, diagonally, in a thickness of 1/4-inch. Drizzle the molasses/mustard sauce over the steal. Use green onions to garnish, as desired. Serve.

Nutrition: Calories: 179 Fat: 4g Carb: 8g Protein: 7g

Lime Coconut Skirt Steak

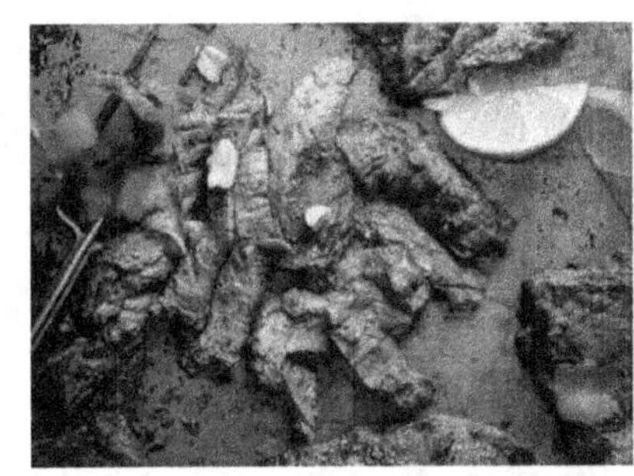

Servings: 4

Preparation time: 4 1/2 hours

Ingredients:

1/2 cup of coconut milk, light

1/4 cup of sugar, coconut

2 tbsp. of lime juice, fresh

2 tsp. of lime zest, fresh

2 tsp. of fish sauce, Thai-flavored

2 tsp. of ginger root, grated

lb. of 4"-cut skirt steak, beef

1/2 tsp. of salt, kosher, coarse

Directions:

Whisk the fish sauce, coconut milk, lime juice, lime zest, ginger and coconut sugar in small sized bowl.

Place the steak in one-gallon sized zipper lock bag. Pour marinade into bag. Press the air out, and then seal the bag. Refrigerate for four to 12 hours. Preheat the grill to high. Drain the steak. Discard the leftover marinade. Pat the steaks dry. Sprinkle with coarse salt. Then oil the grill rack. Place the steaks on grill.Cook for two minutes, then turn steaks 1/4 turn, creating hash marks. Continue cooking for 30-90 more seconds on the first side. Flip the steaks. Continue to cook for two to five minutes till done as you desire.

Allow the steaks to rest for four minutes or longer on your cutting board. Slice across the grain, lengthways. Serve.

Nutrition: Calories: 326 Fat: 24g Carb: 8g Protein: 8g

Pork Chops Butternut Squash

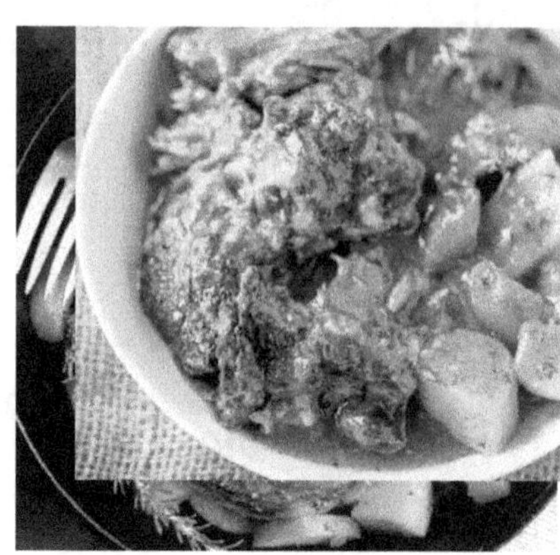

Servings: 4

Preparation time: 1/2 hour

Ingredients:

Nonstick spray

4 x 4-oz. 3/4" thick pork chops, center-cut loin, boneless

1 tsp. of spice blend for pumpkin pie

1/2 tsp. of pepper, black, ground

1/4 tsp. of salt, kosher

1 x 1 1/4-lb. butternut squash - 1 cup of pre-chopped onions, refrigerated

1/4 cup of water, filtered - 1 tbsp. of chopped mint, fresh

Directions: Heat largesized skillet on medhigh. Spray with nonstick spray. Evenly sprinkle the pork with 1/8 tsp. of salt, plus spice and ground pepper. Add the pork to the pan and sauté for three or four minutes on both sides, till done as you desire. Remove the pork out of the pan and keep it warm. Pierce the squash a few times using a fork. Place it onto a few paper towels in your microwave oven. Microwave for 1 minute on HIGH. Peel the squash and halve lengthways. Discard the membrane and seeds and chop the squash coarsely.Use nonstick spray to coat the pan. Add the squash and cover. Cook for seven to eight minutes while occasionally stirring. Add the onion and leave pan uncovered while cooking for five minutes. Stir it frequently. Add 1/4 cup filtered water and cook till the liquid has evaporated. Scrape the pan, loosening any bits that have browned. Remove pan from heat and stir in 1/8 tsp. of kosher salt. Add mint. Evenly spoon the squash mixture over the pork. Serve.

Nutrition: Calories: 606 Fat: 26.4g Carb: 8.3g Protein: 79.8g

Slow Cooker Pot Roast

Servings: 6

Preparation time: 15 minutes + 7 hours slow cooker time

Ingredients:

1 x 8-oz. pkg. of mushrooms, pre-sliced

1 x 8-oz. container of pre-chopped bell pepper, green, refrigerated

Nonstick spray

1/4 cup + 2 tbsp. of ketchup, low sodium

1/4 cup of water, filtered

1 tbsp. of Worcestershire sauce, reduced sodium

1/2 tsp. of pepper, black, ground

1/4 tsp. of salt, kosher

2 lbs. of pot roast, shoulder cut, boneless

Directions:

Coat a medium slow cooker with nonstick spray. Place bell peppers and mushrooms in it.

Combine ketchup, followed by next four ingredients in small sized bowl and stir till blended well.

Heat largesized nonstick skillet on medhigh. Coat the roast and pan using nonstick spray.

Cook roast for three minutes per side, till browned well.

Place roast over the veggies in the slow cooker. Add ketchup mixture. Cover. Cook for an hour on the HIGH setting. Then reduce the heat down to LOW setting and cook for six to seven hours, till roast has become tender. Serve sauce and veggies over the roast.

Nutrition: Calories: 166 Fat: 24g Carb: 8g Protein: 78g

Grilled Sweet Spicy Lamb Chops

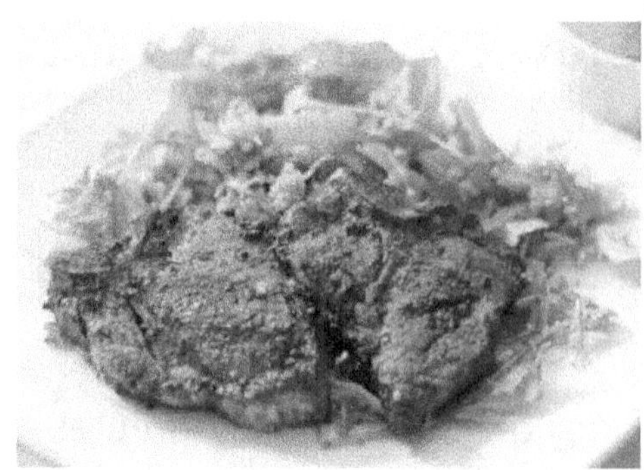

Servings: 4

Preparation time: 15 minutes

Ingredients:

3/4 tsp. of cinnamon, ground

1/2 tsp. of pepper, black, ground

1/4 tsp. of allspice, ground

1/4 tsp. of cumin, ground

1/8 tsp. of salt, kosher

1/8 tsp of red pepper, ground

oz. 1"-thick, trimmed lamb loin chops

Nonstick spray

Optional: lime wedges, fresh

Directions:

Prepare the grill.

Combine the first six ingredients in small sized bowl. Rub this mixture over the lamb evenly.

Spray a grill rack with nonstick spray and place the lamb on it. Grill for four to five minutes per side, till done as you prefer. Place lamb with lime wedges alongside, if you desire, and serve.

Nutrition:

Calories: 126

Fat: 24g

Carb: 9g

Protein: 8g

Steak Pineapple Rice

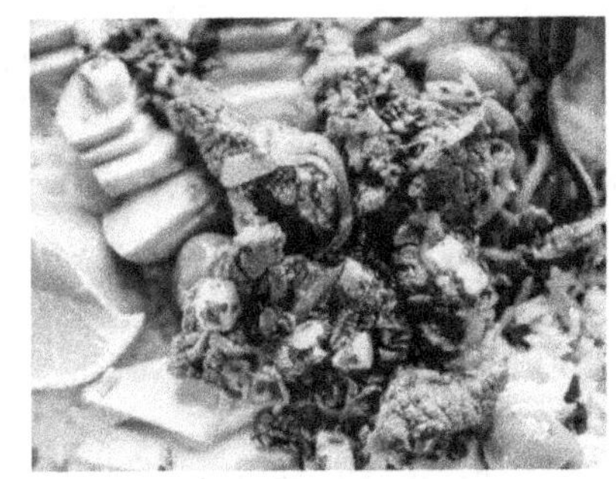

Servings: 4

Preparation time: 1 1/4 hour

Ingredients:

1/4 cup of soy sauce, low sodium

1/2 tsp. of pepper, black

4 x 4-oz. fillets, beef tenderloin

Nonstick spray

1 x 8-oz. can of drained pineapple slices packed in

juice

6 scallions

2 x 8 3/4 oz. pkgs. of brown rice, pre-cooked

3/4 tsp. of salt, kosher, + extra if desired

Directions:

Combine the soy sauce, beef and pepper in large sized zipper top bag. Massage the sauce into the beef. Allow it to sit unrefrigerated for seven or eight minutes. Turn the bag now and then.

As steak is marinating, heat large sized grill pan on medhigh. Use nonstick spray to coat the pan. Arrange the scallions and pineapple in the pan. Cook for five minutes, till the veggies are charred well. Turn so they will char more evenly. Cut the pineapple and scallions into small pieces. Heat the rice using the Directions on the package. Add and stir salt, pineapple and onions. Keep the mixture warm.

Add the beef to the grill pan. Cook for three minutes per side, till done as you desire. Serve over rice mixture.

Nutrition: Calories: 606 Fat: 26.4g Carb: 8.3g Protein: 79.8g

Rosemary Garlic Pork Chops

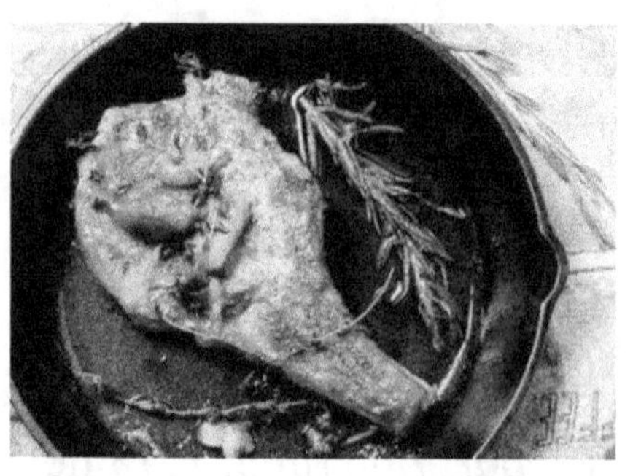

Servings: 4

Preparation time: 45 minutes

Ingredients:

4 loin chops, pork

Salt, kosher

Pepper, black, ground

1 tbsp. of rosemary, minced

2 minced garlic cloves

1 stick of melted butter, unsalted

1 tbsp. of oil, olive

Directions:

Preheat the oven to 375F. Season pork chops as desired.

Mix butter, garlic and rosemary together in small sized bowl and set it aside.

In oven-safe skillet on medhigh, heat the oil and add the pork chops. Sear till they are golden, about four minutes. Flip them, then cook for four more minutes. Generously brush chops with the garlic butter.

Place the skillet in oven. Cook at 375F till cooked completely through, about 8-12 minutes and serve.

Nutrition:

Calories: 236

Fat: 24g

Carb: 13g

Protein: 18g

Balsamic Orange Lamb Chops

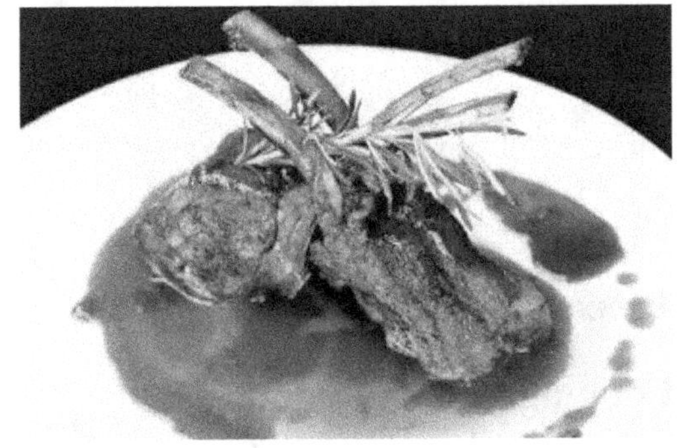

Servings: 4

Preparation time: 55 minutes

Ingredients:

1 tbsp. + 1 tsp. of oil, olive

2 tsp. of orange rind, grated

1 tbsp. of orange juice, fresh

8 x 4-oz. trimmed rib chops, lamb

1 tsp. of salt, kosher

1/2 tsp. of pepper, black, ground

Nonstick spray

3 tbsp. of vinegar, balsamic

Directions:

Combine 1 tbsp. oil with orange juice and rind in largesized, zipper-top bag. Add the lamb. Turn and coat evenly. Allow to sit unrefrigerated for eight to 10 minutes. Remove the lamb from zipper top bag. Evenly sprinkle with kosher salt and ground pepper.

Heat large sized grill pan on medhigh. Use nonstick spray to coat the pan. Add the lamb and cook for two minutes per side till done as you desire.

Pour the vinegar in small-sized skillet on medhigh. Bring to boil. Cook for three minutes, till vinegar has become syrupy. Drizzle remaining 1 tsp. of oil and the vinegar over the lamb. Serve hot.

Nutrition: Calories: 176 Fat: 24g Carb: 3g Protein: 9.8g

Pork Chops with Mushrooms

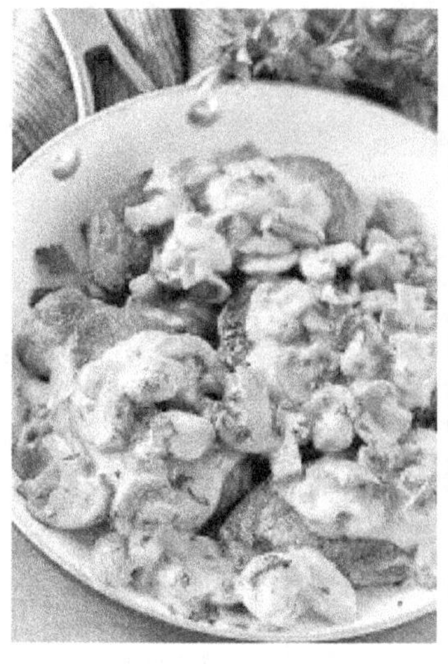

Preparation time: 10 minutes

Cooking time: 40 minutes

Servings: 3

Ingredients

Mushrooms: 8 ounces [sliced].

Garlic powder: 1 tsp.

Onion: 1 chopped

Sugar-free mayonnaise: 1 cup

Pork chops: 3 [boneless].

Ground nutmeg: 1 tsp.

Balsamic vinegar: 1 Tbsp.

Coconut oil: ½ cup

Directions:

Heat coconut oil in a pan.

Add onions, and mushrooms and stir-fry for 4 minutes.

Add pork chops, season with nutmeg, and garlic powder. Brown on both sides.

Place pan in the oven at 350F and bake for 30 minutes.

Transfer pork chops to plates and keeps warm.

Heat the pan over medium heat.

Add mayonnaise and vinegar over mushrooms mixture. Stir well and take off the heat.

Drizzle sauce over pork chops and serve.

Nutrition: Calories: 413 Fat: 82.9g Carb: 7g Protein: 21.7g

Italian Pork Rolls

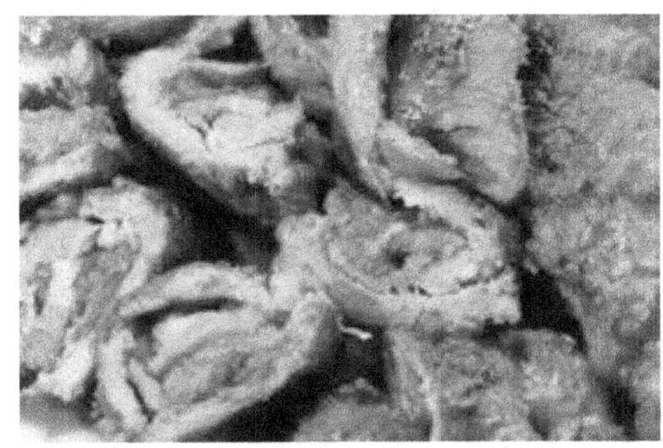

Preparation time: 10 minutes

Cooking time: 20 minutes

Servings: 6

Ingredients

Prosciutto slices: 6

Fresh parsley: 2 Tbsp. [chopped].

Pork cutlets: 1 pound [sliced thin].

Ricotta cheese: 1/3 cup

Coconut oil: 1 Tbsp.

Onion: ¼ cup [chopped].

Garlic: 3 cloves [minced].

Parmesan cheese: 2 Tbsp. [grated].

Canned diced tomatoes: 15 ounces

Chicken stock: 1/3 cup

Salt and ground black pepper to taste - Italian seasoning: ½ tsp.

Directions: Use a meat pounder to flatten pork pieces. Place prosciutto slices on top of each piece then, divide ricotta cheese, parsley, and parmesan cheese.   Roll each pork piece and secure with a toothpick. Heat coconut oil in a pan. Add pork rolls, cook until brown on both sides, and transfer to a plate. Heat the pan again over medium heat, and garlic and onion. Stir-fry for 5 minutes. Add stock and cook for 3 minutes. Discard toothpicks from pork rolls and return to the pan. Add tomatoes, salt, pepper, Italian seasoning. Stir and bring to a boil. Lower heat, cover the pan and cook for 30 minutes.   Serve.

Nutrition: Calories: 256 Fat: 13.6g Carb: 5.7g Protein: 17.2g

Thai Beef

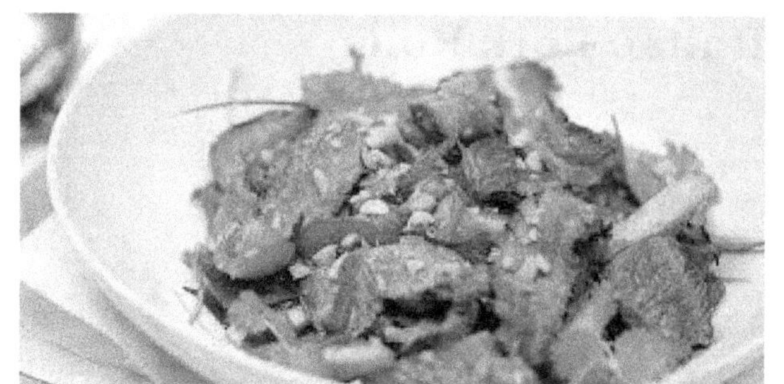

Preparation time: 10 minutes

Cooking time: 10 minutes

Servings: 6

Ingredients

Beef stock: 1 cup

Peanut butter: 4 Tbsp.

Garlic powder: ¼ tsp.

Onion powder: ¼ tsp.

Coconut aminos: 1 Tbsp.

Lemon pepper: 1 ½ tsp.

Beefsteak: 1 pound [cut into stripes].

Salt and ground black pepper to taste

Green bell pepper: 1 [seeded and chopped].

Green onions: 3 [chopped].

Directions:

In a bowl, mix peanut butter with stock, aminos, lemon pepper. Stir well and set aside.

Heat a pan on medium heat.

Add beef, season with salt, pepper, onion, garlic powder, and cook for 7 minutes.

Add green pepper. Stir-fry for 3 minutes.

Add green onions and peanut sauce. Stir and cook for 1 minute.

Serve.

Nutrition: Calories: 222 Fat: 10.3g Carb: 5.9g Protein: 26.6g

Beef Pot Roast

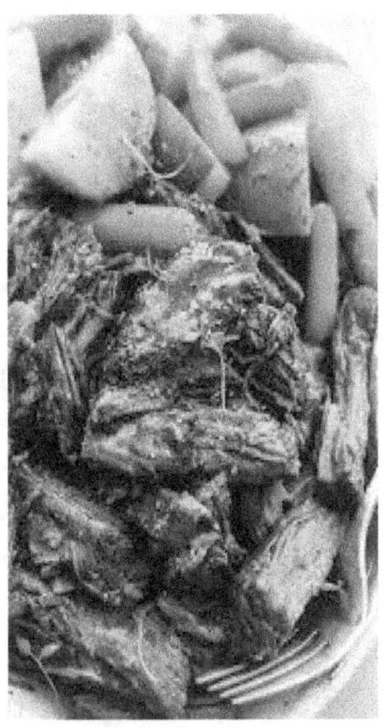

Preparation time: 10 minutes

Cooking time: 1 hour 15 minutes

Servings: 4

Ingredients

Beef roast: 3 ½ pounds

Mushrooms: 4 ounces [sliced].

Beef stock: 12 ounces

Onion powder: 1 ounce

Olive oil: ½ cup

Directions:

In a bowl, mix stock with onion powder, olive oil, and mix.

Put beef roast in a pan.

Add mushrooms, stock mixture, and cover with aluminum foil.

Place in an oven at 300F and bake for 1 hour and 15 minutes.

Allow roast to cool, slice, and serve with the gravy on top.

Nutrition:

Calories: 990

Fat: 50.3g

Carb: 6.7g

Protein: 123g

Glazed Beef Meatloaf

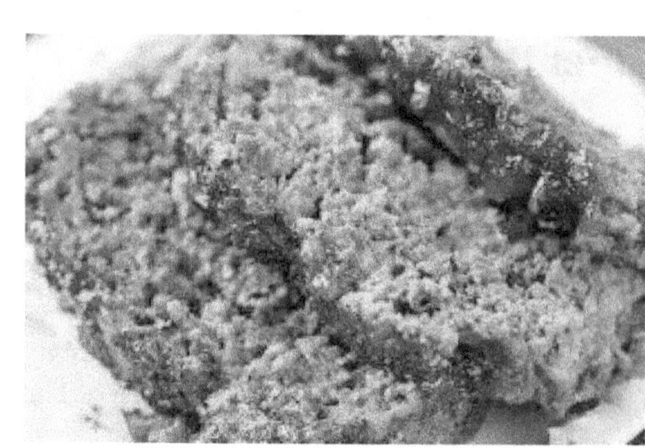

Preparation time: 10 minutes

Cooking time: 1 hour 10 minutes

Servings: 6

Ingredients

White mushrooms: 1 cup [chopped].

Ground beef: 3 pounds

Fresh parsley: 2 Tbsp. [chopped].

Garlic cloves: 2 [minced].

Onion: ½ cup [chopped].

Red bell pepper: ¼ cup [chopped].

Almond flour: ½ cup

Parmesan cheese: 1/3 cup [grated].

Eggs: 3

Salt and ground black pepper to taste

Balsamic vinegar: 1 tsp.

For the glaze: Swerve: 1 Tbsp. - Tomato paste: 2 Tbsp. - Balsamic vinegar: 2 cups

Directions: In a bowl, mix beef with eggs, salt, pepper, 1 tsp. vinegar, Parmesan cheese, almond flour, parsley, bell pepper, onion, garlic, and mushrooms. Transfer into a loaf pan and bake in the oven at 375F for 30 minutes.   Heat a small pan over medium heat.   Add tomato paste, swerve, and 2 cups vinegar. Stir well and cook for 20 minutes.   Take the meatloaf out of the oven. And spread the glaze on meatloaf.   Place in the oven at the same temperature and bake for 20 minutes.   Cool, slice, and serve.

Nutrition: Calories: 606 Fat: 26.4g Carb: 8.3g Protein: 79.8g

Beef with Tzatziki

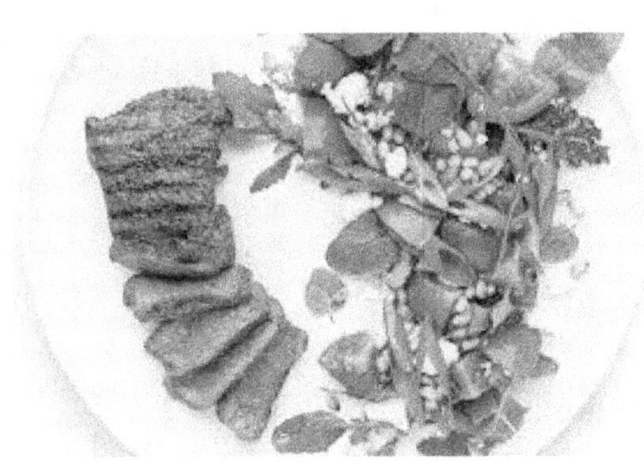

Preparation time: 10 minutes

Cooking time: 15 minutes

Servings: 6

Ingredients

Almond milk: ¼ cup

Ground beef: 17 ounces

Onion: 1 [grated].

Cauliflower rice: 5 oz.   - Egg: 1 [whisked].

Fresh parsley: ¼ cup [chopped].

Salt and ground black pepper to taste

Garlic: 2 cloves, minced - Fresh mint: ¼ cup [chopped].

Dried oregano: 2 ½ tsp. - Olive oil: ¼ cup

Cherry tomatoes: 7 ounces [cut in half].

Cucumber: 1 [sliced thin].

Baby spinach: 1 cup

Lemon juice: 1 ½ tbsp. - Jarred tzatziki: 7 ounces

Directions:Put the cauliflower rice in a bowl. Add milk, and set aside for 3 minutes. Drain, add beef, egg, salt, pepper, oregano, mint, parsley, garlic, onion. Stir well. Shape balls from mixture and place on a work surface. Heat a pan with half of the oil over medium heat. Add meatballs and cook for 8 minutes. Stir to cook all around. Transfer them to a tray. In a bowl, mix spinach with tomato and cucumber. Add meatballs, remaining oil, salt, pepper, and lemon juice. Add tzatziki and toss to coat. Serve.

Nutrition: Calories: 322 Fat: 18.6g Carb: 9.9g Protein: 29.2g

Meatballs with Mushroom Sauce

Preparation time: 10 minutes

Cooking time: 25 minutes

Servings: 6

Ingredients

Ground beef: 2 pounds

Salt and black pepper to taste

Garlic powder: ½ tsp.

Coconut amions: 1 Tbsp.

Beef stock: ¼ cup

Almond flour: ¾ cup - Fresh parsley: 1 Tbsp. [chopped].

Dried onion flakes: 1 Tbsp.

For the sauce: Onion: 1 cup [chopped]. - Mushrooms: 2 cups [sliced].

Bacon fat: 2 Tbsp. - Butte: 2 Tbsp. - Coconut aminos: ½ tsp.

Sour cream: ¼ cup - Beef stock: ½ cup

Salt and ground black pepper to taste

Directions: In a bowl, mix beef with salt, pepper, garlic powder, 1 tbsp. coconut aminos, ¼ cup beef stock, almond flour, parsley, and onion flakes. Stir well and shape 6 meatballs. Place them on a baking sheet. Place in an oven at 375F and bake for 18 minutes. Heat butter in a pan and add bacon fat over medium heat. Add mushrooms, stir, and cook for 4 minutes. Add onions, stir, and cook for 4 minutes. Add ½ tsp. coconut anions, sour cream, and ½ cup beef stock. Stir well and bring to a simmer. Remove from heat, and adjust seasoning. Stir well. Divide the beef meatballs between plates and serve with mushroom sauce on top.

Nutrition: Calories: 452 Fat: 23.5g Carb: 4.9g Protein: 53.2g

Ground Beef Casserole

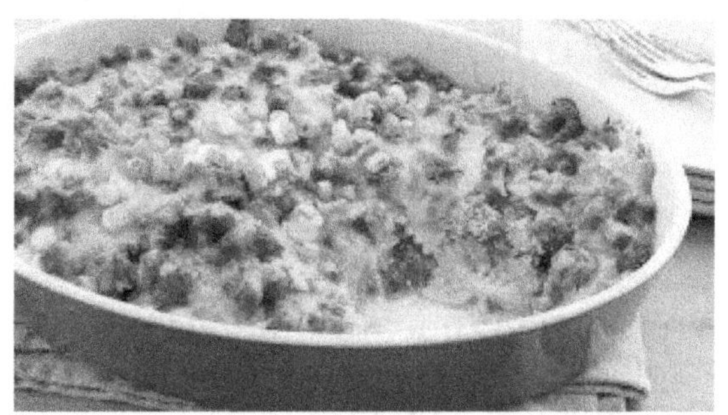

Preparation time: 10 minutes

Cooking time: 35 minutes

Servings: 6

Ingredients

Onion flakes: 2 tsp.

Worcestershire sauce: 1 Tbsp.

Ground beef: 2 pounds

Garlic: 2 cloves [minced].

Salt and ground black pepper to taste

Mozzarella cheese: 1 cup [shredded].

Cheddar cheese: 2 cups [shredded].

Keto mayonnaise: ½ cup

Sesame seeds: 2 Tbsp. [toasted].

Dill pickle: 20 slices

Romaine lettuce heat: 1, torn

Directions:

In a pan, add beef, onion flakes, Worcestershire sauce, salt, pepper, and garlic. Stir-fry for 5 minutes. Transfer to a baking dish. Add 1 cup cheddar cheese, mozzarella cheese, and half of the mayonnaise. Stir and spread evenly. Arrange pickle slices on top. Sprinkle remaining cheddar and sesame seeds. Place in an oven at 350F and bake for 20 minutes. Turn oven to broil and bake the casserole for 5 minutes. Divide lettuce on plates. Top with a beef casserole and the remaining mayonnaise. Serve.

Nutrition: Calories: 577 Fat: 36.1g Carb: 4.8g Protein: 57.6g

Zucchini Noodles and Beef

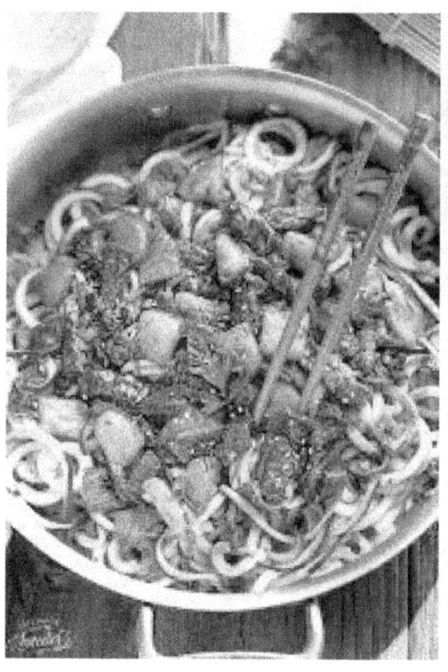

Preparation time: 10 minutes

Cooking time: 20 minutes

Servings: 5

Ingredients

Ground beef: 1 pound

Onion: 1 [chopped].

Garlic: 2 cloves [minced].

Canned diced tomatoes: 14 ounces

Dried rosemary: 1 Tbsp.

Dried sage: 1 Tbsp.

Dried oregano: 1 Tbsp.

Dried basil: 1 Tbsp.

Dried marjoram: 1 Tbsp.

Salt and black pepper to taste

Zucchinis: 2 [cut with a spiralizer].

Directions:

Heat a pan over medium heat.

Add garlic and onion. Stir and brown for 2 minutes.

Add beef, stir and cook for 6 minutes.

Add tomatoes, salt, pepper, rosemary, sage, oregano, marjoram, and basil. Stir and simmer for 15 minutes.   Divide zucchini noodles into bowls and add the beef mixture.   Serve.

Nutrition: Calories: 206 Fat: 6g Carb: 8.2g Protein: 29.5g

Lamb Salad

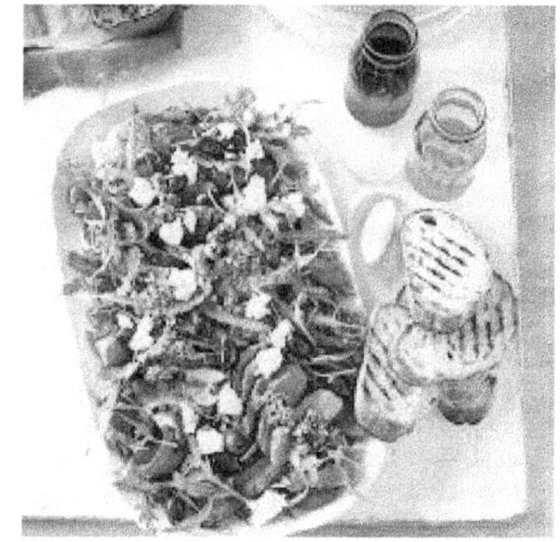

Preparation time: 10 minutes

Cooking time: 35 minutes

Servings: 4

Ingredients

Olive oil: 1 Tbsp.

Leg of lamb: 3 pounds [bone removed and leg butterflied].

Salt and ground black pepper to taste

Cumin: 1 tsp.

A pinch of dried thyme

Garlic: 2 cloves [minced].

For the salad:

Feta cheese: 4 ounces [crumbled].

Pecans: ½ cup

Spinach: 2 cups - Lemon juice: 1 ½ Tbsp.

Olive oil: ¼ cup - Fresh mint -1 cup [chopped].

Directions:Rub lamb with salt, pepper, 1 Tbsp. oil, thyme, cumin, and minced garlic. Place on a preheated grill pan over medium-high heat and cook for 40 minutes: flipping once. Spread pecans on a lined baking sheet. Place in an oven at 350F and toast for 10 minutes. Transfer grilled lamb to a cutting board, set aside to cool down, and slice. In a salad bowl, mix spinach with 1 cup mint, feta cheese, ¼ cup olive oil, lemon juice, toasted pecans, salt, pepper and toss to coat. Add lamb slices on top and serve.

Nutrition: Calories: 431 Fat: 52.5g Carb: 8.3g Protein: 67.3g

Philly Cheese Steak Pockets

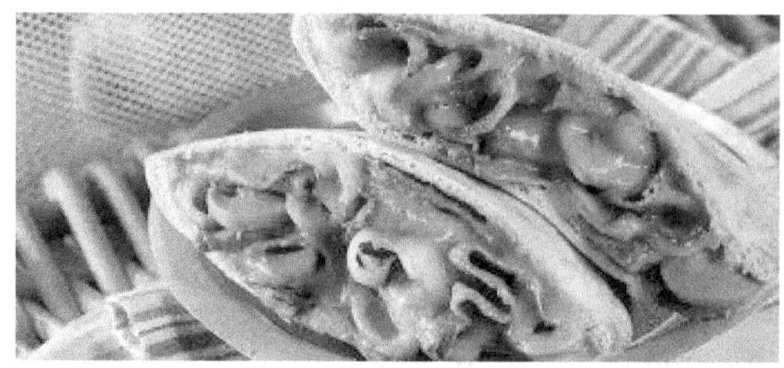

Servings: 4

Preparation time: 40 minutes

Ingredients:

1 pound of sliced flank steak

2 sliced bell peppers

1/2 sliced onion

2 minced garlic cloves

2 tbsp. of seasoning blend, Italian

2 tbsp. of oil, olive

Salt, kosher

Pepper, ground

4 slices of provolone cheese

Directions:

Heat your grill for medhigh heat.

Toss steak, olive oil, Italian seasoning, garlic, onion and peppers together. Season as desired.

Place the steak mixture in individual foil packets. Fold the packs up. Grill for 10 minutes, to cook meat through.

Open the packets and add the provolone cheese. Cover the grill and cook for two minutes to melt the cheese. Remove and serve.

Nutrition: Calories: 606 Fat: 26.4g Carb: 8.3g Protein: 79.8g

Keto smoky bacon meatballs

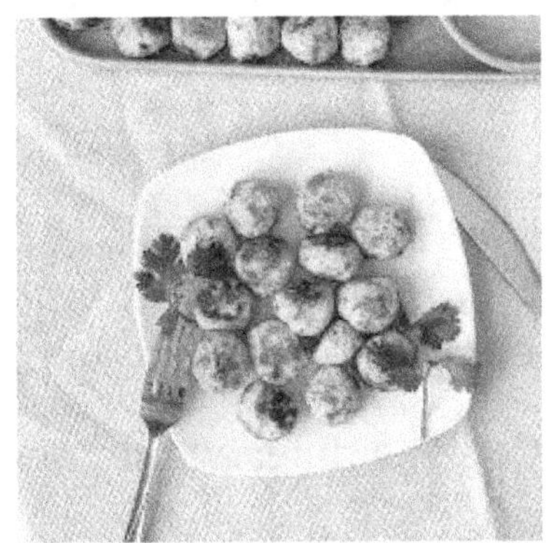

Preparation time: 10 minutes

Cooking time: 20 minutes

Servings: 6

INGREDIENTS

2 chicken breasts or 1-pound (450 g) ground chicken

8 strips of bacon, fried and crumbled

1 potato, whisked

2 cloves of garlic, peeled

1 teaspoon (7 g) onion powder

2 drops of liquid smoke

4 teaspoons (60 ml) of avocado or olive oil.

Directions:

Place everything (except oil) in a food processor and mix well.

Shape 20-24 tiny meatballs from the mixture.

Put the oil in a large pan and fry the meatballs until the meat is cooked (cover one side for 5 minutes until browned, then turn over and cook the other side for 5-10 minutes until done). You're probably going to have to cook in a couple of pots.

Nutrition:

Calories: 606

Fat: 26.4g

Carb: 8.3g

Protein: 79.8g

Keto steak saute

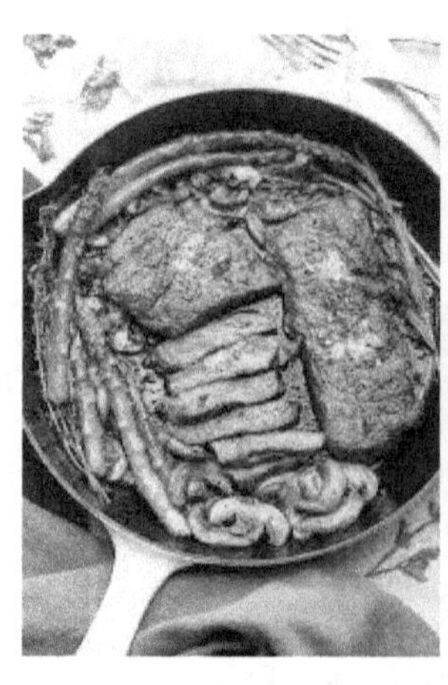

Preparation time: 10 minutes

Cooking time: 20 minutes

Servings: 6

Ingredients:

1 beef steak, diced

1/2 onion, peeled and sliced

2 cloves of garlic, minced 2 teaspoons (30 ml) of avocado oil, to be prepared with

 Directions:

1.Add the avocado oil to the pan and sauté the steak, onion and garlic.

NOTES: All dietary information are calculated and focused on the volume of each meal. Carbs Net: 6 g

Nutrition:

Calories: 236

Fat: 26.4g

Carb: 8.3g

Protein: 79.8g

Barbecued Trout Cooked in Newspaper

Preparation time: 10 minutes

Cooking time: 40 minutes

Servings: 3

Ingredients:6 pounds wild sea trout Salt to taste.

Directions:

Scale the wild sea trout, remove the gills, guts, eyes, and proceed to wash.

Pat with a kitchen towel everywhere ensuring there are no running drips.

Make diagonal cuts on the sides and sprinkle salt into these cuts.

Wrap the trout using multiple newspaper layers ensuring that it is completely sealed.

Secure the newspapers with a butcher's string and submerge the trout in cold water. The reason why you need to soak the package is to wet the newspaper.

Prepare your package of a hot barbeque and proceed to cook for 40 minutes occasionally flipping until ready.

Remove the fish from the barbeque and allow it to sit for a few minutes.

Proceed to cut the butcher's string and remove the newspaper. Place on a tray and flake off the flesh using a fork.

Enjoy your trout.

Tip: You will experience excessive smoking as the water from the newspaper. However, the experience is worthwhile as the fish will thoroughly steam inside. Additionally, when flaking the fish ensure you get rid of all the bones.

Calories per serving: 408

Nutrition: Calories: 230 Fat: 24g Carb: 3g Protein: 8g

Smoked Lamb Ribs on the Grill

Preparation Time: 5 minutes

Cooking Time: 2 hours 35 minutes

Servings: 2

Ingredients

8 lamb rib chops1 tablespoon butter1 tbsp salt Pinch of black pepper

Directions:

Rub your lamb chops with salt and black pepper on all the sides.

In the meantime, prepare your smoker for indirect heating. When ready, place the ribs on the cooler part of the smoker ensuring no direct contact with the fire, cover, and wait for 1 hour.

After 1 hour, remove the ribs and wrap using a foil.

Return them meat-side-down and continue cooking for 35 minutes on low heat ensuring. Flip and cook for 30 more minutes. Remove from the smoker and allow the ribs to rest for 30 minutes then unwrap.

Take your tongue on a tasty tour

Calories per serving: 383 Kcal

Nutrition:

Calories: 236

Fat: 14g

Carb: 13g

Protein: 18g

Skinny Steaks

Preparation Time: 2 hours

Cooking Time: 10 minutes

Servings: 2

Ingredients:

2 pounds of fatty beef sirloin, sliced into 2-inch strips Salt and pepper to taste

Directions:

Sprinkle the beef strip with salt and pepper. Proceed to dry bring in a refrigerator for 2 hours.

After the 2 hours remove from the fridge and pat dry with paper towels.

Heat your grill to screaming hot temperatures without closing the lid. In case you are using charcoal, ensure the coals are piled high enough. If it's a gas grill, lower the grate closer to the burner.

Place the meat on the hottest grill part occasionally flipping to cool the hot surface, reduce heat build-up, and to prevent the meat interior from overcooking. The idea is to aim for 130° F in the middle uniform and a dark brown exterior with no grill marks.

Tip: If you are working with steaks measuring 1 inch thick or less, ensure you flip every minute.

Calories per serving: 121.0 Kcal

Nutrition:

Calories: 129

Fat: 21g

Carb: 13g

Protein: 18g

T-bone Grilled Steak

Preparation Time: 40 minutes, 1-4 hours chilling

 Cooking Time: 15-20 minutes

Servings: 4-6

Ingredients:

4-6 T-bone steaks

2 tbsp sea salt

Rub

1 tsp thyme1 tbsp onion powder1 tsp garlic powder1 tsp cayenne pepper2 tbsp coriander seeds
Directions:

Mix dry spices and grind

Rub the steaks and salt to your taste.

Set to the refrigerator to chill for 1-4 hours.

Heat your grill, place the steaks on it and cook 2 min each side several times.

Check the meat temperature. For the medium rare it should be 125 degrees.

Serve in 5-7 minutes

Calories per serving: 3 ounce T-bone steak has 210 Kcal

Nutrition:

Calories: 128

Fat: 24g

Carb: 18g

Protein: 18g

Slow Cooked Texas-Style Pulled Pork

Preparation time: 10 Minutes

Cooking time: 7 hours

Servings: 8

Ingredients:

4 lbs pork shoulder roast1/2 cup chicken brothCeltic sea salt.

A spoonful of butter.

Directions:

Place the pork roast in a slow cooker, add the butter, salt, and the broth.

Cover the cooker and proceed to cook for 7 hours on low.

After 7 hours, remove and leave to sit for 5 minutes.

Depending on what you like, shred the pork with your hands or a fork.

Return the shredded pork to the crockpot and lightly stir until the meat is covered in juices.

Serve.

Calories per serving: 530 Kcal

Nutrition:

Calories: 198

Fat: 20g

Carb: 13g

Protein: 18g

Pork Rind and Chicken

Preparation time: 10 minutes

Cooking time: 30 minutes

Servings: 3

Ingredients

300 g chicken breastI bag of ground pork rinds2 eggs2 tablespoons butterSalt

Directions:

Season your chicken with salt.

In a bowl, crack and whip the eggs for the batter.

Proceed to thinly spread the pork crumbs on a flat plate.

Dip the seasoned breasts in the beaten egg bowl and shake to remove the excess liquid.

Depending on your preferred cooking method, pan sear or bake the chicken.

When ready, remove and spread the butter and rebake for 15 more minutes.

Once golden brown, your meal is ready for serving.

Calories per serving: 290 Kcal

Nutrition:

Calories: 167

Fat: 21g

Carb: 19g

Protein: 18g

Ground Beef

Preparation time: 10 minutes

Cooking time: 15 minutes Serves: 4

Ingredients

½ lb Ground beef1 tbsp butter

½ tsp salt

 Directions:

On a flaming hot frying pan, add butter and gently place your ground beef.

Sear for 10 minutes and reduce the heat to medium-high heat.

Continue to sear for 5 minutes and add salt.

Serve on a plate and enjoy!

Calories per serving: 127 kcal

Nutrition:

Calories: 36

Fat: 14g

Carb: 8.3g

Protein: 18g

Shredded Chicken and Bacon

Preparation time: 10 minutes

Cooking time: 5 hours 15 minutes

Servings: 1

Ingredients:

1 chicken breast slow cooked1 slice bacon chopped2 tablespoon butter1 tablespoon salt1 tablespoon black pepper

Directions:

First, cook your chicken in a slow cooker for 5 hours. When ready, shred using your hands or a fork.

Pan fry the bacon using butter. When it starts producing fats, add the shredded chicken and cook for 5 minutes.

Add more flavor with salt and pepper.

Serve and enjoy.

Calories per serving: 390.6 Kcal

Nutrition:

Calories: 606

Fat: 26.4g

Carb: 8.3g

Protein: 79.8g

Southern Slow Steak

Preparation time: 15 minutes

Cooking time: 8 hrs

Servings: 8

Ingredients:

2 pounds sirloin steaks, chopped into 3" pieces1 teaspoon salt to taste1 teaspoon pepper taste5 tablespoons butter1/2 cup beef broth3 cups of water

Directions:

Sprinkle your steak pieces with salt and pepper.

Add butter on a large pan and heat over high. Once hot enough add your steaks.

Continue cooking until they brown on each side.

Remove from the pan and place them in your crockpot.

Add 3 cups of water in the frying pan together with the broth and reduce the heat to medium-high. Bring to a boil.

Pour the mixture in your crockpot, cover, and cook for 8 hours on low.

Once fork tender, your meal is ready to be served.

Calories per serving: 275 kcal

Nutrition:

Calories: 189

Fat: 14g

Carb: 3g

Protein: 18g

Chapter 10: Poultry

Salt and Pepper Turkey

Preparation time: 10 minutes

Cooking time: 20 minutes

Servings: 6

Ingredients

1 whole turkey of about 9 -10 pounds, discard giblets

3-5 tablespoons butter

Coarse salt to taste

Freshly ground pepper to taste

Serves: 5-8

Directions:

Pour 2 cups water in a large roasting pan. Place a rack in the pan. Start at the neck and loosen the skin on the breast area. Take some of the butter and rub it beneath the skin. Sprinkle salt and pepper, generously all over the turkey and the cavity. Using a thick kitchen string, tie up the legs together. Place turkey on the rack and tuck the wings below. Bake in a preheated oven at 350 ° F for 2-3 hours or until the internal temperature when checked with an instant read thermometer in the thickest part of the meat shows 165 ° F. Baste the turkey with remaining butter after every 25 to 30 minutes. Slightly shake the turkey so that the cooked juice falls into the pan. Remove turkey from the oven and place on your cutting board. Tent with foil and let it sit for 30 minutes. When cool enough to handle, cut into slices. Drizzle some of the cooked liquid from the pan over the turkey and serve.

Nutrition: Calories: 189 Fat: 24g Carb: 8.3g Protein: 9.8g

Turkey in Cream Sauce

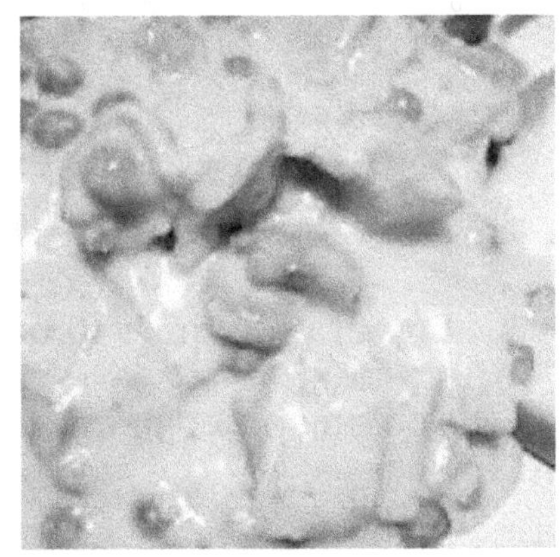

Preparation time: 10 minutes

Cooking time: 20 minutes

Servings: 6

Ingredients

3 tablespoons butter

¾ cup heavy cream

Salt to taste

Pepper to taste

¾ cup chicken stock

2 cups cooked, chopped turkey

Serves: 4

Directions:

Place a large pan over medium heat. Add butter and cook until it turns golden in color.

Add stock and simmer for 5-6 minutes.

Add cream, turkey, salt and pepper. Simmer for a few minutes.

Serve hot.

Nutrition:

Calories: 178

Fat: 34g

Carb: 33g

Protein: 18g

Turkey with Cheddar Cheese Sauce

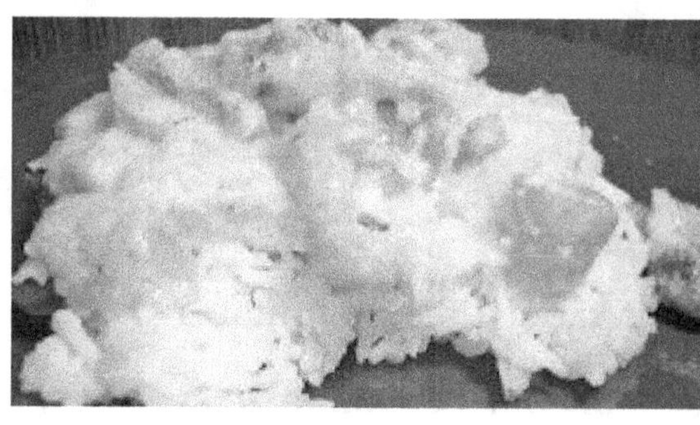

Preparation time: 10 minutes

Cooking time: 30 minutes

Servings: 6

Ingredients

4 slices (1 ounce each) cooked turkey breast

2 tablespoons butter + extra to grease

½ cup milk or half and half

Pepper to taste

Salt to taste

½ cup shredded cheddar cheese

Directions:

Take a small square baking dish of about 6x6 inches and grease with a little butter.

Lay the turkey slices in the dish.

Place a saucepan over medium heat. Add butter and melt.

Add turkey, salt, pepper and simmer for a couple of minutes.

Add cheese and cook until it melts and well blended with the other ingredients.

Turn off the heat.

Pour over the turkey.

Bake in a preheated oven at 350 ° F for about 20 minutes or until the sauce is bubbling.

Nutrition: Calories: 606 Fat: 26.4g Carb: 8.3g Protein: 79.8g

Duck Leg Confit

Preparation time: 10 minutes

Cooking time: 20 minutes

Servings: 6

Ingredients

2 duck legs with thigh, trimmed of excess fat and retain it

3-5 tablespoons butter

Table salt to taste

½ tablespoon kosher salt

Freshly ground pepper to taste

2 cups duck fat (that was retained)

¾ teaspoon whole peppercorns

Directions: Place the duck legs on a large plate, with the skin side facing down. Season with kosher salt and pepper. Pour the duck fat in a baking dish. Stack the duck legs in the baking dish and place in the refrigerator for 10 to 12 hours. Remove the duck and rinse in cold water. Lightly wipe off the salt and pepper. Dry with paper towels. Remove the duck fat and place in an enameled cast iron pot. Scatter peppercorns on the fat. Sprinkle salt over it. Place the duck, with the skin side facing down in the pot. Place some duck fat on top of the duck. Cover and place in a preheated oven. Bake at 350 ° F for about 2-3 hours or until the meat falls away from the bone. Strain the fat from the dish into a bowl. Retain the fat to store meat or use in some other recipe. If you want to serve right away, transfer the duck legs into a pan, with the skin side facing down. Place the pan over medium high heat and sear until the skin is crisp and brown. If you want to eat after a few days, remove the meat from the bones and keep it in a stoneware container. Pour some of the retained fat over the meat. (Fat should cover by at least ¼ inch over the meat). Place the container in the refrigerator until use. It can last for a month.

Nutrition: Calories: 178 Fat: 34g Carb: 23g Protein: 58g

Italian Chicken

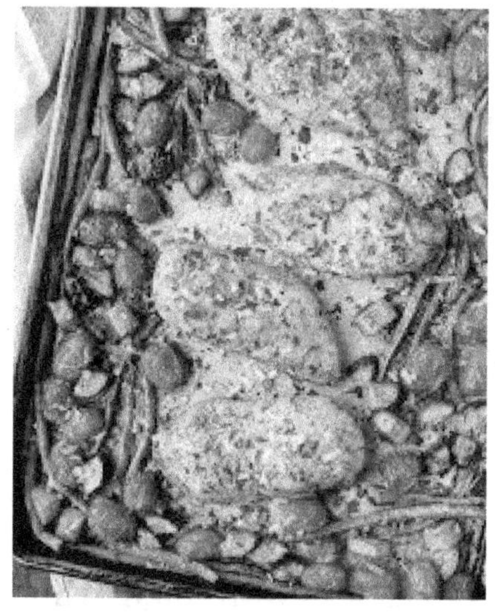

Preparation time: 10 minutes

Cooking time: 20 minutes

Servings: 4

Ingredients

Olive oil: ¼ cup

Onion: 1 [chopped].

Chicken breasts: 4 [skinless and boneless].

Garlic: 4 cloves [minced].

Salt and ground black pepper to taste

Green olives: ½ cup [pitted and chopped].

Anchovy fillets: 4 [chopped].

Capers: 1 Tbsp. [chopped].

Tomatoes: 1 pound [chopped].

Red chili flakes: ½ tsp.

Directions:

Season chicken with salt, pepper, and rub with half of the oil.

Place into a preheated pan over high heat.

Cook for 2 minutes, flip, and cook for 2 minutes. Place chicken breasts in the oven at 450F and bake for 8 minutes. Take chicken out of the oven and divide between the plates. Heat the same pan with remaining oil.

Add olives, garlic, onion, anchovies, chili flakes, capers, stir. Cook for 1 minute. Add salt, pepper, tomatoes, and stir-fry for 2 minutes. Drizzle over chicken breasts and serve.

Nutrition: Calories: 533 Fat: 37.1g Carb: 9.8g Protein: 57.5g

DIY Orange Chicken

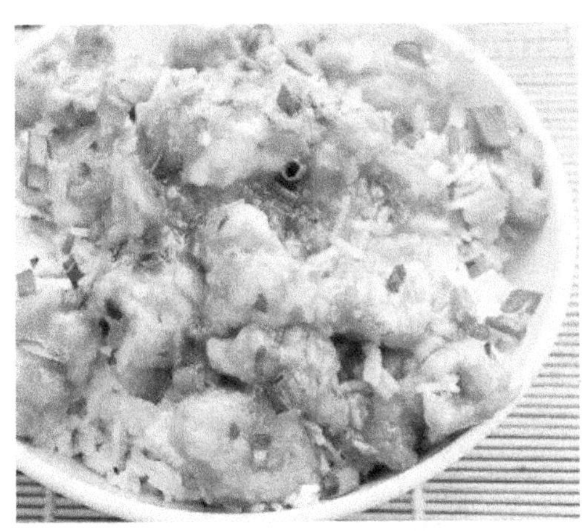

Servings: 4

Preparation time: 3/4 hour

Ingredients:

2 cups of flour, all-purpose

2 beaten eggs, large

2 cups of breadcrumbs, panko

1 pound of chunk-cut chicken breasts, skinless,

boneless

Salt, kosher

Pepper, ground

2 fresh oranges– zest and juice only

1/3 cup of soy sauce, low sodium - 1/4 cup of honey, organic

2 minced garlic cloves - 2 tsp. of ginger, grated

2 tbsp. of corn starch - 2 cups of jasmine rice, cooked

For garnishing: Sesame seeds - Green onions, sliced

Directions: Set up dredging station using a bowl of flour, a bowl of eggs and a bowl of bread crumbs. Dredge chicken first in flour. Then coat it with the eggs and cover with bread crumbs. Season as desired. Line a cookie sheet with baking paper. Arrange the chicken on it. Bake till it isn't pink anymore, which usually takes 17-20 minutes or so.To prepare the sauce, combine soy sauce, orange juice, honey, corn starch, garlic and ginger in small sized pan on med. heat. Whisk till combined well. Cook till it thickens, usually five or six minutes.Transfer the chicken to large sized bowl. Toss it in the orange sauce and coat well. Serve on rice with green onions, orange zest and sesame seeds.

Nutrition: Calories: 606 Fat: 26.4g Carb: 8.3g Protein: 79.8g

Chicken Fajitas

Preparation time: 10 minutes

Cooking time: 15 minutes

Servings: 4

Ingredients

Chicken breasts: 2 pounds [skinless, boneless, and cut into strips].

Garlic powder: 1 tsp.

Chili powder: 1 tsp.

Cumin: 2 tsp.

Lime juice: 2 Tbsp.

Salt and black pepper to taste

Sweet paprika: 1 tsp.

Coconut oil: 2 Tbsp. - Coriander: 1 tsp.

Green bell pepper: 1 [seeded and sliced].

Red bell pepper: 1 [seeded and sliced]. - Onion - 1 [sliced].

Fresh cilantro: 1 Tbsp. [chopped]. - Avocado: 1 [sliced].

Limes: 2 [cut into wedges].

Directions: In a bowl, mix lime juice with coriander, paprika, garlic powder, pepper, salt, cumin, and chili powder. Add chicken pieces and toss to coat. Heat half of the oil in a pan. Add chicken and cook for 3 minutes on each side. Transfer to a bowl. Heat the pan with remaining oil. Add onion and bell peppers, stir. Cook for 6 minutes. Return chicken to pan. Add more salt, pepper, and mix. Divide on plates. Top with avocados, lime wedges, cilantro, and serve.

Nutrition: Calories: 443 Fat: 34g Carb: 7.2g Protein: 48.1g

Skillet Chicken and Mushrooms

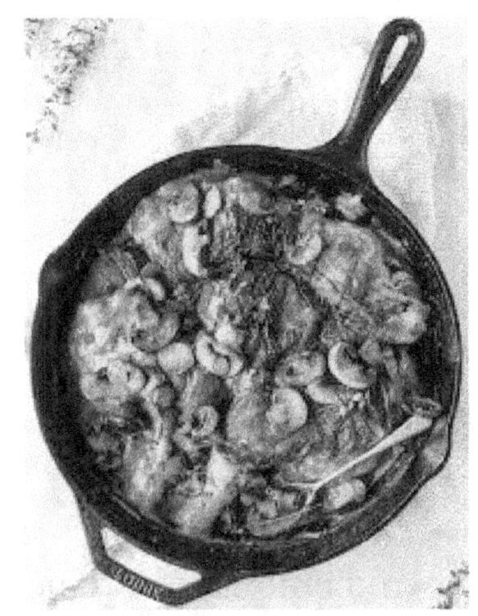

Preparation time: 10 minutes

Cooking time: 30 minutes Se

Servings: 4

Ingredients

Chicken thighs: 4

Mushrooms: 2 cups [sliced].

Butter: ¼ cup

Salt and ground black pepper to taste

Onion powder: ½ tsp.

Garlic powder: ½ tsp.

Water: ½ cup

Dijon mustard: 1 tsp.

Fresh tarragon: 1 Tbsp. [chopped].

Directions:

Heat half of the butter in a pan.

Add chicken thighs, season with salt, pepper, garlic powder, and onion powder.

Cook for 3 minutes on each side and transfer to a bowl.

Heat the same pan with remaining butter.

Add mushrooms, stir, and cook for 5 minutes. Add mustard and water. Stir well. Return chicken pieces to the pan, stir, cover, and cook for 15 minutes. Add the tarragon and stir. Cook for 5 minutes. Serve.

Nutrition: Calories: 664 Fat: 33.3g Carb: 1.2g Protein: 85.7g

Crock Pot Chicken Gizzards and Hearts

Preparation time: 10 minutes

Cooking time: 10 hours

Servings: 6

Ingredients:1 bag of chicken gizzards1 bag chicken hearts8 cups beef brothCeltic sea salt and pepper to taste Preparation

Rinse the chicken parts in water.

Place them in a slow cooker with the gizzards going first followed by hearts.

Add salt and pepper

In goes the beef broth.

Cover and cook for 10 hours.

Calories per serving: 663 Kcal

Nutrition:

Calories: 324

Fat: 26.4g

Carb: 8.3g

Protein: 79.8g

Pan-Seared Duck Breast

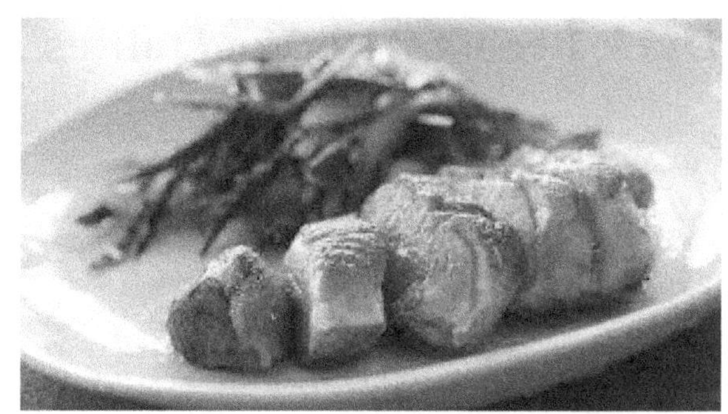

Preparation time: 10 minutes

Cooking time: 20 minutes

Servings: 1

Ingredients

Duck breast: 1 medium [skin scored].

Swerve: 1 Tbsp.

Heavy cream: 1 Tbsp.

Butter: 2 Tbsp.

Orange zest: ½ tsp.

Salt and ground black pepper to taste

Baby spinach: 1 cup

Fresh sage: ¼ tsp.

Directions:

Heat butter in a pan.

Add swerve and stir until the butter browns.

Add orange zest and sage. Stir and cook for 2 minutes.

Add heavy cream and stir again. Heat another pan over medium heat. Add duck breast, skin side down and cook for 4 minutes. Flip and cook for another 3 minutes. Pour orange sauce over duck breast, stir, and cook for a few minutes. Add spinach to the pan with the sauce, stir and cook for 1 minute.

Take duck off heat, slice duck breast, and arrange on a plate. Drizzle orange sauce on top and serve with the spinach on the slide.

Nutrition: Calories: 588 Fat: 54.3g Carb: 6.6g Protein: 42.2g

Duck Breast with Vegetables

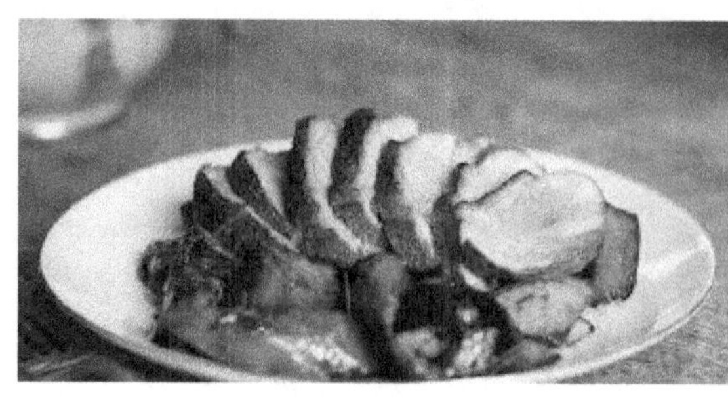

Preparation time: 10 minutes

Cooking time: 10 minutes

Servings: 2

Ingredients

Duck breasts: 2 [skin on and sliced thin].

Zucchini: 2, sliced

Coconut oil: 1 Tbsp.

Green onion: 1 bunch [chopped].

Daikon: 1 [chopped].

Green bell peppers: 2 [seeded and chopped].

Salt and ground black pepper to taste

Directions:

Heat coconut oil in a pan.

Add green onions and stir-fry for 2 minutes.

Add bell peppers, daikon, zucchini, salt, and pepper. Cook for 10 minutes.

Heat another pan over medium heat.

Add duck slices, cook for 3 minutes on each side. Transfer to a pan with vegetables.

Cook for 3 minutes, divide on plates and serve.

Nutrition: Calories: 188 Fat: 20.3g Carb: 3g Protein: 5.2g

Duck Breast Salad

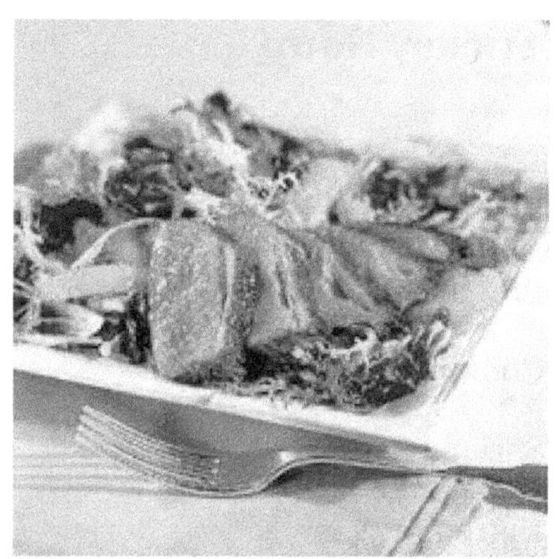

Preparation time: 10 minutes

Cooking time: 15 minutes

Servings: 4

Ingredients

Swerve: 1 Tbsp.

Shallot: 1 [peeled and chopped].

Red vinegar: ¼ cup

Olive oil: ¼ cup

Water: ¼ cup - Raspberries: ¾ cup

Dijon mustard: 1 Tbsp.

Salt and ground black pepper to taste

For the salad: Baby spinach: 10 ounces

Duck breasts: 2 medium [boneless].

Goat cheese: 4 ounces [crumbled].

Salt and ground black pepper to taste

Raspberries: 2 cups - Pecans halves: ½ cup

Directions:In a blender, mix the swerve, with shallot, vinegar, water, oil, ¾ cup raspberries, mustard, salt, pepper. Blend well. Strain into a bowl and set aside. Score duck breast, season with salt, pepper, and place skin side down into a pan heated over medium-high heat. Cook for 8 minutes, flip, and cook for 5 minutes. Divide spinach on plates sprinkle the goat cheese, pecan halves, and 2 cups raspberries. Slice duck breasts and add on top of raspberries. Drizzle raspberries vinaigrette on top and serve.

Nutrition: Calories: 628 Fat: 52g Carb: 5.1g Protein: 32g

Turkey Soup

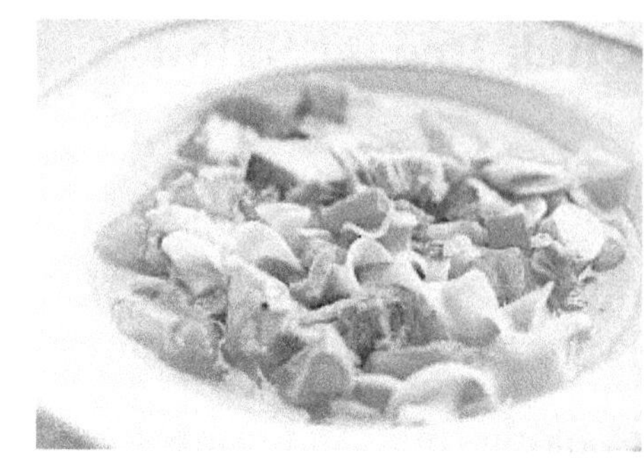

Preparation time: 10 minutes

Cooking time: 30 minutes

Servings: 4

Ingredients

Celery: 3 stalks [chopped].

Onion: 1 [chopped].

Butter - 1 Tbsp.

Turkey stock: 6 cups

Salt and ground black pepper to taste

Fresh parsley: ¼ cup, chopped

Baked spaghetti squash: 3 cups [chopped].

Turkey: 3 cups [cooked and shredded].

Directions:

Heat butter in a pot.

Add celery and onion. Stir-fry for 5 minutes.

Add turkey meat, stock, parsley, salt, and pepper. Stir-fry for 20 minutes.

Add spaghetti squash, stir, and cook soup for 10 minutes.

Serve.

Nutrition: Calories: 272 Fat: 8.5g Carb: 3.7g Protein: 33.6g

Turkey Chili

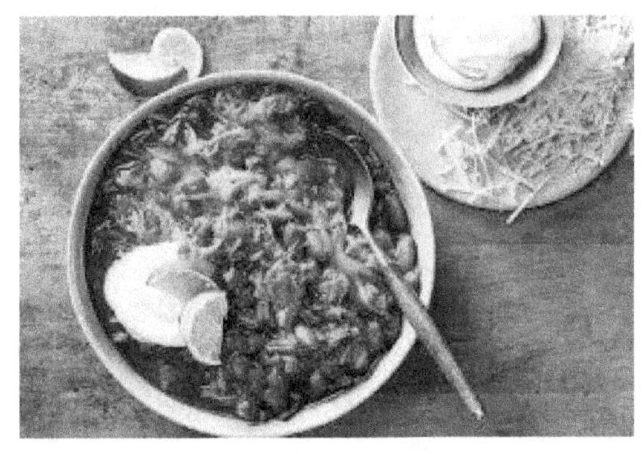

Preparation time: 10 minutes

Cooking time: 20 minutes

Servings: 8

Ingredients

Turkey meat: 4 cups [cooked and shredded].

Squash: 2 cups [cooked].

Chicken stock: 6 cups

Salt and ground black pepper to taste

Canned chipotle peppers: 1 Tbsp. [chopped].

Garlic powder - ½ tsp.

Salsa verde: ½ cup

Coriander: 1 tsp.

Cumin: 2 tsp.

Sour cream: ¼ cup

Fresh cilantro: 1 Tbsp. [chopped].

Directions:

Heat the stock in a pan over medium heat.

Add squash, stir, and cook for 10 minutes.

Add turkey, salt, pepper, coriander, cumin, salsa verde, garlic powder, and chipotles. Stir and cook for 10 minutes.

Add sour cream, stir, take off heat, and divide into bowls. Top with some chopped cilantro and serve.

Nutrition: Calories: 153 Fat: 5.6g Carb: 2.9g Protein: 21.9g

Turkey and Tomato Curry

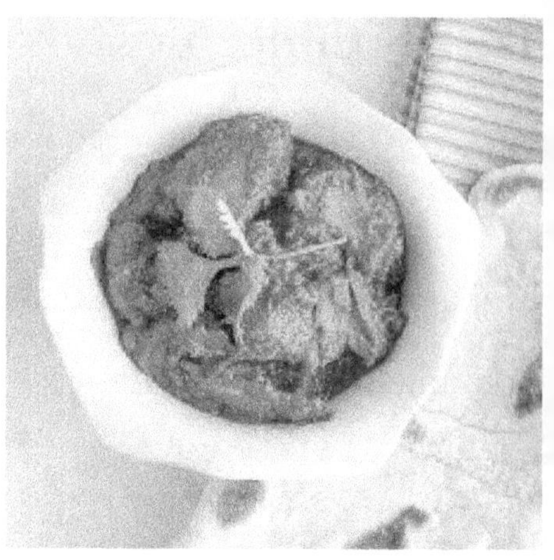

Preparation time: 10 minutes

Cooking time: 20 minutes

Servings: 4

Ingredients

Turkey meat: 18 ounces [minced].

Spinach: 3 ounces

Canned diced tomatoes: 20 ounces

Coconut oil: 2 Tbsp.

Coconut cream: 2 Tbsp.

Garlic: 2 cloves [minced].

Onions: 2 [sliced].

Coriander: 1 Tbsp.

Fresh ginger: 2 Tbsp. [grated].

Turmeric: 1 Tbsp.

Cumin: 1 Tbsp.

Salt and ground black pepper to taste

Chili powder: 2 Tbsp.

Directions: Heat coconut oil in a pan. Add onion and stir-fry for 5 minutes. Add ginger and garlic. Stir-fry for 1 minute.

Add chili powder, turmeric, cumin, coriander, salt, pepper, and tomatoes. Stir. Add coconut cream, stir, and cook for 10 minutes. Remove from heat. Blend with a hand mixer and mix with spinach and turkey meat. Bring to a simmer, cook for 15 minutes. Serve.

Nutrition: Calories: 240 Fat: 4g Carb: 2g Protein: 12g

Stuffed Chicken Breast

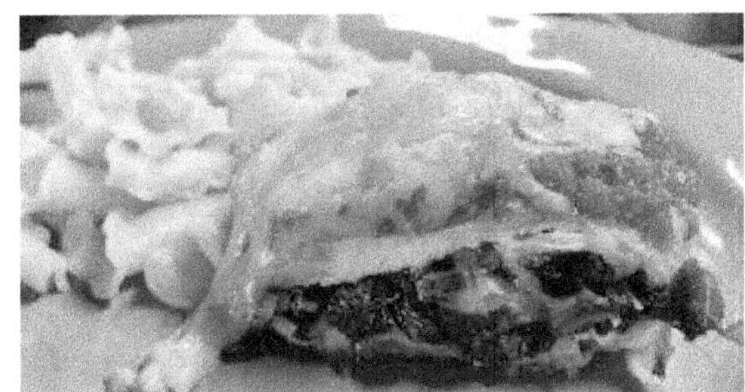

Preparation time: 10 minutes

Cooking time: 15 minutes

Servings: 3

Ingredients

Spinach: 8 ounces [cooked and chopped].

Chicken breasts - 3

Salt and ground black pepper to taste

Cream cheese: 4 ounces [softened]

Feta cheese: 3 ounces [crumbled]

Garlic: 1 clove [minced].

Coconut oil: 1 Tbsp.

Directions:

In a bowl, mix feta cheese with cream cheese, garlic, salt, pepper, and spinach. Stir well.

Place chicken breasts on a work surface.

Cut a pocket in each, stuff them with spinach mixture, and season them with some salt and pepper.

Heat coconut oil in a pan.

Add stuffed chicken, and cook for 5 minutes on each side.

Place in the oven for 450F.

Bake for 10 minutes.

Serve.

Nutrition: Calories: 412 Fat: 49.3g Carb: 5.2g Protein: 57.2g

Chicken Casserole

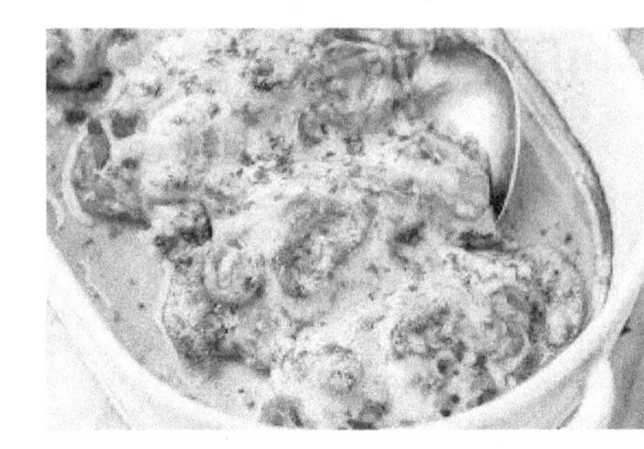

Preparation time: 10 minutes

Cooking time: 40 minutes

Servings: 8

Ingredients

Chicken breast: 1 ½ pound [skinless, boneless, and cubed].

Egg: 1

Almond flour - 1 cup

Parmesan cheese: ¼ cup [grated]

Dried parsley: 1 ½ tsp.

Avocado oil: 4 Tbsp.

Spaghetti squash: 4 cups [cooked].

Mozzarella cheese: 6 ounces [shredded].

Tomato paste: 1 ½ cups - Minced Garlic: 1 tsp.   - Dried basil: 1 tsp.

Dried rosemary: ½ tsp. - Fresh basil for serving

Directions: In a bowl, mix almond flour with parmesan, salt, pepper, garlic powder, 1 tsp. parsley. Stir. In another bowl, whisk the egg with a pinch of salt and pepper. Dip chicken in egg and then in almond flour mixture. Heat a pan with 3 tbsp. oil over medium-high heat. Add chicken and cook until they are golden brown on both sides, and transfer to paper towels.   In a bowl, mix spaghetti squash with salt, pepper, dried basil, 1 tbsp. oil and remaining parsley. Stir. Spread this mixture into a dish, add chicken pieces, and then tomato paste, minced garlic, dried rosemary and dried basil. Top with shredded mozzarella cheese. Place in the oven at 375F and bake for 30 minutes.   Sprinkle with fresh basil at the end, set the casserole aside to cool. Serve.

Nutrition: Calories: 622 Fat: 16.3g Carb: 8.1g Protein: 57

Chicken-Stuffed Peppers

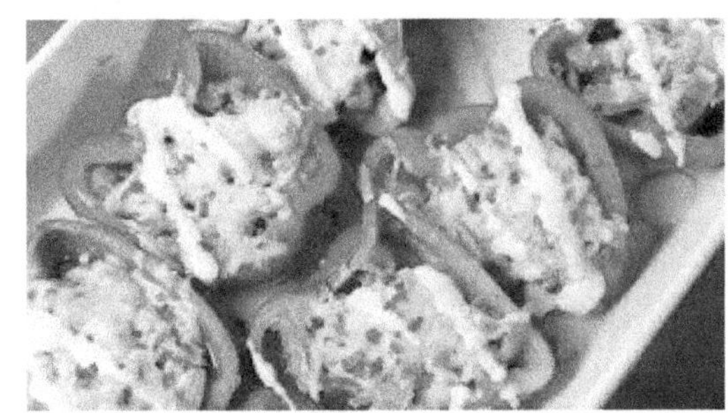

Preparation time: 10 minutes

Cooking time: 40 minutes

Servings: 3

Ingredients

Cauliflower florets: 2 cups

Salt and ground black pepper to taste

Onion: 1 [chopped].

Chicken breasts: 2 [skinless, boneless, cooked, and shredded].

Fajita seasoning: 2 Tbsp.

Butter: 1 Tbsp.

Bell peppers: 6 [tops cut off and seeds removed].

Water: 2/3 cup

Directions:

Put cauliflower florets in a food processor. Add a pinch of salt and pepper. Pulse well and transfer to a bowl.

Heat butter in a pan.

Add onions and stir-fry for 2 minutes.

Add cauliflower and stir-fry for 3 minutes.

Add chicken, water, seasoning, salt, pepper. Stir-fry for 2 minutes.

Place bell peppers on a lined baking sheet and stuff each with chicken mixture. Place in an oven at 350F and bake for 30 minutes. Serve.

Nutrition: Calories: 532 Fat: 19g Carb: 5.7g Protein: 60.5g

Crispy Chicken Thighs

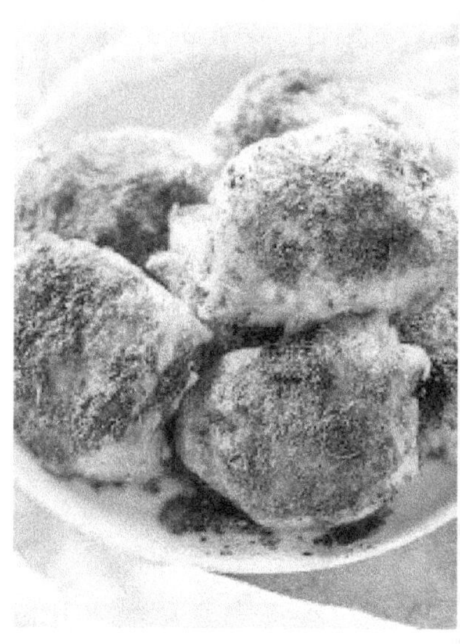

Ingredients

6 chicken thighs, with skin

2 tablespoons butter or lard, melted

Freshly ground pepper to taste

Kosher salt to taste

Serves: 4-8

Preparation

Dry the chicken by patting with paper towels. Season with salt and pepper.

Toss well.

Place the chicken pieces on a baking sheet with the skin side facing up, in a single layer. Drizzle butter over it

Roast in a preheated oven at 400 ° F for 20: 30 minutes or until cooked through. The internal temperature in the thickest part of the meat should show 165 ° F.

If you want the skin to be crisp, broil for a couple of minutes.

Nutrition:

Calories: 606

Fat: 26.4g

Carb: 8.3g

Protein: 79.8g

BBQ Chicken Livers and Hearts

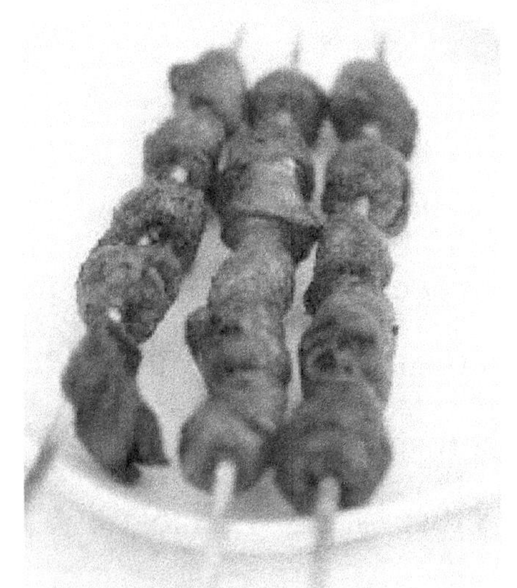

Ingredients

2 pounds chicken livers, thawed to room temperature

2 pounds chicken hearts, thawed to room temperature

Pepper to taste

Salt to taste

A few bamboo skewers, soaked in water for an hour

Serves: 4-6

Preparation

Clear the excess fat from the hearts and livers and clean them too.

Place them flat, in a flexible grilling basket.

Sprinkle salt and pepper over the meat.

Grill on a charcoal grill until the way you like it cooked.

Nutrition:

Calories: 178

Fat: 20g

Carb: 9g

Protein: 68g

Lime Honey Chicken Skewers

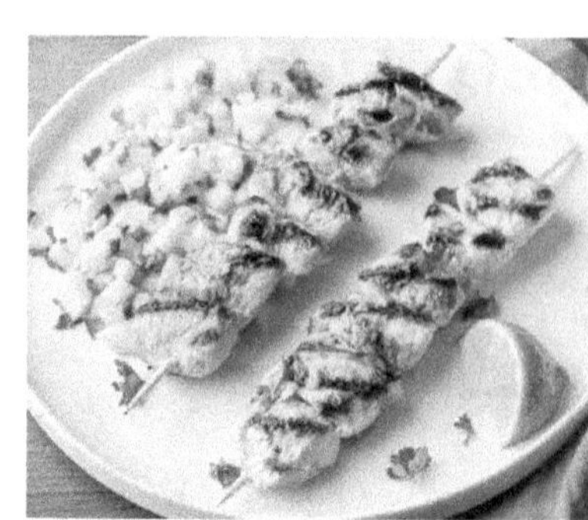

Servings: 4

Preparation time: 35 minutes + 1-hour marinating time

3 tbsp. of soy sauce, low sodium

2 tbsp. of honey, pure

1 tbsp. of oil, vegetable

1 fresh lime, juice only

2 minced cloves of garlic

1 to 2 tsp. of sriracha

Pepper flakes, red, as desired

2 tbsp. of cilantro

1 lb. of chicken breasts, boneless, skinless

Directions:

Combine ingredients up to and including cilantro in small sized bowl. Mix well.

Pour this marinade over the chicken and turn the pieces to coat them. Cover. Allow meat to marinate for an hour or more.

Grill over medhigh for six to eight minutes each side till juices are running clear. Skewer the veggies and chicken. Serve.

Nutrition:

Calories: 26

Fat: 44g

Carb: 3g

Protein: 18g

Chicken with Cheesy Sauce

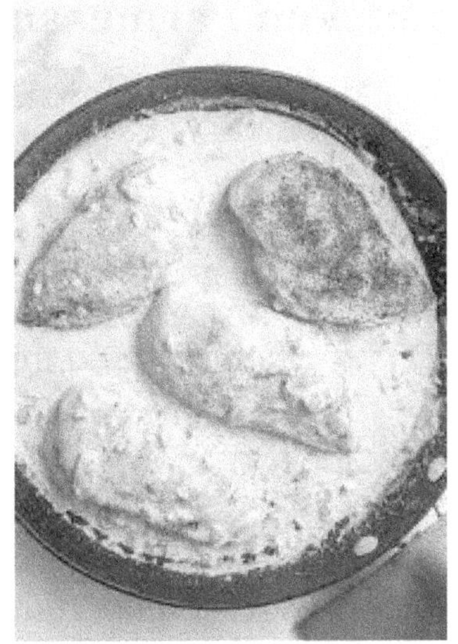

Ingredients

6 chicken thighs

½ teaspoon pepper

½ teaspoon salt

1 cup of chicken bone broth

4 ounces cream cheese

½ cup heavy cream

10 tablespoons butter, divided

1 cup mozzarella cheese, shredded

Serves: 3

Preparation

Place a large skillet over medium heat. Add 2 tablespoons butter and allow it to melt.

Sprinkle salt and pepper over the chicken. Sprinkle beneath the skin also.

Place chicken in the skillet with the skin side facing down.

Cover and cook for 6 minutes or until the skin side is brown. Remove chicken with a slotted spoon and set aside on a plate. Pour broth into the skillet. Scrape the bottom of the pan to remove any browned bits that may be stuck. Add chicken back into the pan. Cover and cook until chicken is cooked through. Meanwhile, make the sauce as follows: Add cream cheese, cream and remaining butter into a saucepan. Place saucepan over low heat. Stir constantly until the mixture is well incorporated. Turn off the heat.

Whisk in the mozzarella cheese. Stir constantly until cheese melts. Place chicken in bowls. Pour cheesy sauce over it and serve.

Nutrition: Calories: 138 Fat: 4g Carb: 8g Protein: 8g

Chicken Parmesan Quinoa

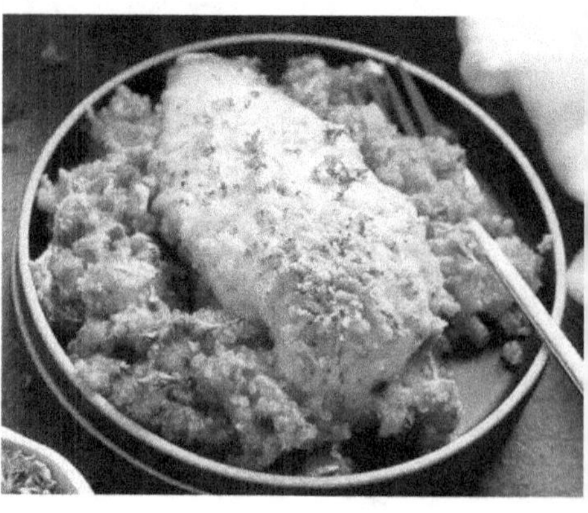

Servings: 4

Preparation time: 50 minutes

Ingredients:

1 cup of quinoa

1 tbsp. of seasoning, Italian

2 halved crossways chicken breasts, skinless,

boneless

Salt, kosher pepper, ground, as desired

1/2 cup of flour, all-purpose

2 beaten eggs, large

1/2 cup of mozzarella cheese shreds

1/4 cup of Parmesan cheese, grated

1 cup of marinara sauce, store bought

Directions:

Preheat the oven to 400F. Oil one cookie sheet lightly.

In 1 1/2 cups of filtered water in large sized sauce pan, cook the quinoa using directions on the package. Add and stir Italian seasoning mix. Season the chicken as desired.

Work in batches to dredge the chicken in the flour, then dip it into the eggs, then dredge it in the quinoa mixture. Be sure to press a bit so the coating sticks. Place the chicken on cookie sheet prepared above. Bake in 400F oven for 18-25 minutes, till chicken is golden brown in color.Top chicken with both cheeses, then the marinara sauce. Place chicken back in oven. Bake till cheeses melt, or about five to seven minutes more. Serve promptly.

Nutrition: Calories: 60 Fat: 9.4g Carb: 3g Protein: 18g

Buffalo Chicken Wraps

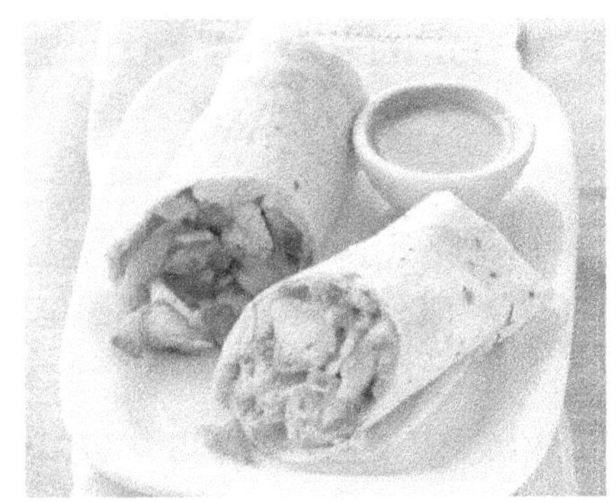

Servings: 4-6

Preparation time: 2 hours

Ingredients:

1 1/2 lbs. of cubed chicken breast, skinless, boneless

1/2 cup of buffalo sauce + extra to drizzle at end, as desired

2 cups of breadcrumbs, plain

4 to 6 soft lettuce leaves

1 cup of quinoa, cooked

1/2 cup of tomatoes, diced

1/2 cup of avocado, diced

For garnishing:

Green onions

Ranch or blue cheese dressing

Directions:

Preheat oven to 375F. Grease a cookie sheet lightly.

Toss chicken into buffalo sauce. Cover the bowl. Refrigerate for 1/2 hour or more.

Pour bread crumbs in shallow dish. Coat chicken pieces evenly. Place on cookie sheet prepared above. It will be crowded, but that's alright.

Bake the chicken for 1/2 hour. You may toss baked chicken in extra buffalo sauce, as desired.

For assembling wraps, fill leaves with quinoa, avocado and tomatoes. Top them using buffalo chicken cubes. Drizzle with dressing. Sprinkle with onions. Serve.

Nutrition: Calories: 189 Fat: 20g Carb: 80g Protein: 7.8g

Taco Turkey Wraps

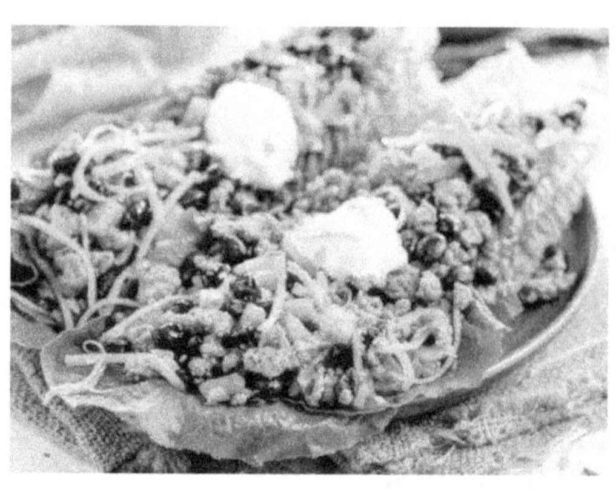

Servings: 4

Preparation time: 25 minutes

Ingredients:

1 tbsp. oil, olive

3/4 cup chopped onion, yellow

1 pound ground turkey, 95% lean

2 garlic cloves

Kosher salt ground pepper

1 tbsp. chili powder

1 tsp. cumin, ground

1/2 tsp. paprika, smoked

1/2 cup tomato sauce, reduced-sodium

1/2 cup chicken broth, low-sodium

To serve: Doubled-up lettuce leaves, Romaine or iceberg

Mexican cheese mix shreds

Diced tomatoes, Roma - Chopped onion, red - Cilantro, chopped

Avocado, diced - Sour cream, light

Directions: Heat oil in skillet on medhigh. Add the onion. Sauté for two minutes. Add the garlic, then the turkey. Season as desired. Cook while tossing and breaking turkey up, for about five minutes, till it has cooked through. Add the chicken broth, tomato sauce, paprika, cumin and chili powder. Reduce to simmer. Cook for five to six minutes till sauce has been reduced. Serve the mixture on lettuce leaves, with any toppings desired.

Nutrition: Calories: 190 Fat: 64g Carb: 8g Protein: 8g

Salt and Pepper Roast Chicken

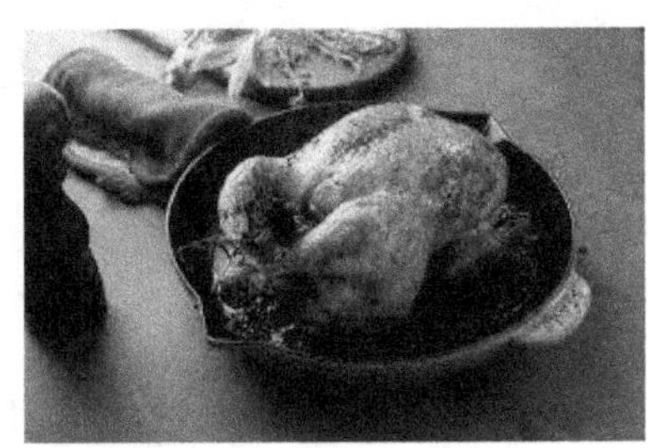

Ingredients

2-3 pounds chicken, cut into parts (bone-in and skin on if using chicken breasts)

Freshly ground pepper to taste

Kosher salt to taste

Serves: 4-8

Preparation

Dry the chicken by patting with paper towels. You can also use whole chicken. Place in a bowl.

Sprinkle salt and pepper over the chicken. Chill for 1-8 hours.

Place the chicken pieces in a roasting pan, with the skin side facing up, in a single layer.

Roast in a preheated oven at 400 ° F for about 30 minutes (or 50-60 minutes if using whole chicken) or until cooked through. The internal temperature in the thickest part of the meat should show 165 ° F.

If you want the skin to be crisp, broil for a couple of minutes.

If using whole chicken, remove from the oven and cool for a while. Slice and serve.

Nutrition:

Calories: 189

Fat: 20g

Carb: 23g

Protein: 9.8g

Parmesan Crusted Chicken Thighs with Bacon Cream Sauce

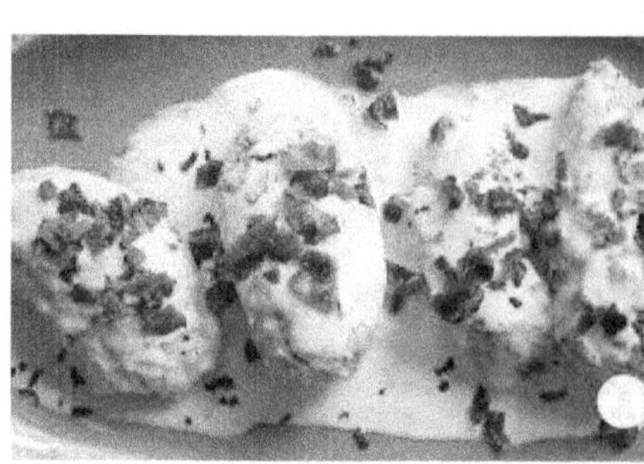

Preparation time: 10 minutes

Cooking time: 20 minutes

Servings: 6

Ingredients:

For Parmesan crusted chicken:

4 chicken thighs

½ cup freshly grated paran cheese¼ teaspoon salt

2 -3 tablespoons butter, melted

¼ teaspoon pepper (optional)

For bacon cream sauce: 3 slices bacon

½ tablespoon sour cream - ¼ cup heavy whipping cream

½ tablespoon shredded parmesan cheese

Serves: 2

Preparation: Add melted butter in a shallow bowl. Place salt, pepper and Parmesan cheese on a plate. Mix well. Dip a chicken thigh in butter. Shake to drop off excess butter. Dredge in the Parmesan and place in a greased

baking dish with the skin side facing up. Repeat with the remaining chicken thighs. Bake in a preheated oven at 400 ° F for about 35-50 minutes depending on the size of the thighs. For bacon cream sauce: Place a skillet over medium heat. Add bacon and cook until crisp. Remove with a slotted spoon (retain the bacon fat in the pan) and set aside on a plate. When cool enough to handle, crumble the bacon. Add cream into the skillet and whisk until well blended. Continue whisking until tiny bubbles appear on the edges of the pan. Whisk in the sour cream. Divide the chicken into 2 plates. Divide the sauce among the plates and serve.

Nutrition: Calories: 187 Fat: 24g Carb: 23g Protein: 9.8g

Simple, Pan-fried Chicken Breasts

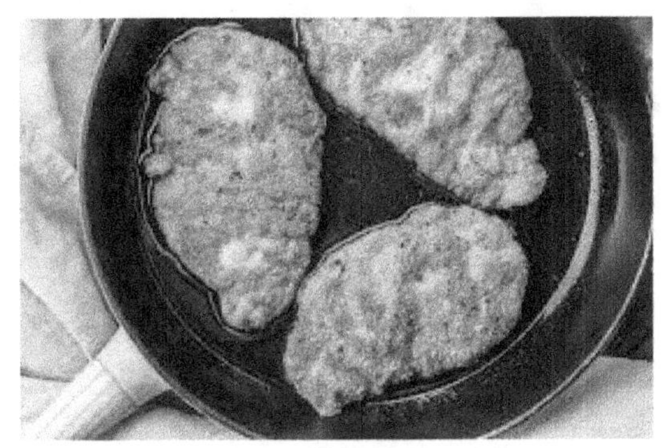

Preparation time: 10 minutes

Cooking time: 40 minutes

Servings: 6

Ingredients

8 chicken breast halves

2 tablespoons butter or lard

Freshly ground pepper to taste

Kosher salt to taste

¼ cup grated parmesan cheese (optional)

Serves: 4-5

Preparation

Place a stainless steel or cast: iron skillet over medium heat. Add butter or lard and let the pan heat.

Using a meat mallet, pound the chicken breast until the chicken is uniformly thick.

Season with salt and pepper if using. Let it rest for 15-20 minutes.

Place an ovenproof skillet over high heat. Place chicken in the skillet.

Cook for 2-3 minutes without stirring or covering. Cook until golden brown and the fat is released. Flip sides cook for 2-3 minutes.

Remove from the heat and garnish with Parmesan cheese.

Broil for 2-3 minutes and serve.

Nutrition: Calories: 129 Fat: 24g Carb: 23g Protein: 9.8g

Chicken with Creamy Bacon Sauce

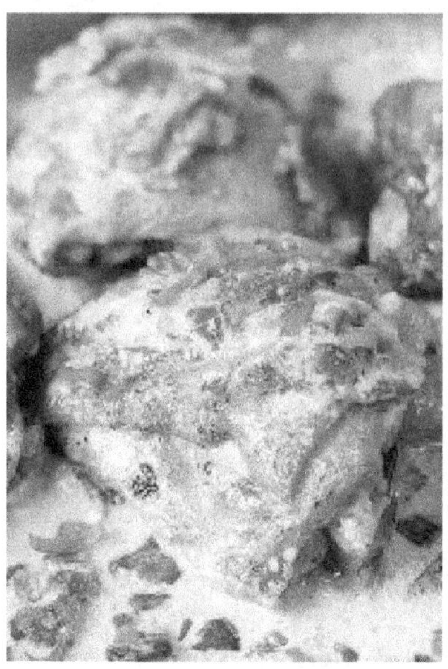

Preparation time: 5 minutes

Cooking time: 30 minutes

Servings: 4

Ingredients

10 chicken thighs

½ teaspoon pepper

½ teaspoon salt

1 cup of chicken bone broth

1 cup double heavy cream

4 tablespoons butter, softened - 16 slices bacon

Serves: 10

Preparation: Place a pan over medium heat. Add bacon and cook until brown. Drain the fat remaining in the pan. When cool enough to handle, chop into small pieces. Set aside. Place a large skillet over medium heat. Add butter and melt. Sprinkle salt and pepper over the chicken. Sprinkle beneath the skin as well. Place chicken in the skillet with the skin side facing down. Cover and cook for 6 minutes or until the skin side is brown. Remove chicken with a slotted spoon and set aside on a plate. Pour broth into the skillet. Scrape the bottom of the pan to remove any browned bits that may be stuck. Add chicken back into the pan. Add half the bacon. Cover and cook until chicken is cooked through. Remove chicken with a slotted spoon and set aside. Add cream and remaining butter into the same skillet. Stir constantly until the mixture is well incorporated. Add chicken back into the skillet and mix well. Simmer for a couple of minutes. Turn off the heat. Place chicken in bowls. Sprinkle remaining bacon on top and serve.

Nutrition: Calories: 600 Fat: 26.4g Carb: 8.3g Protein: 79.8g

Easy Chicken Salad

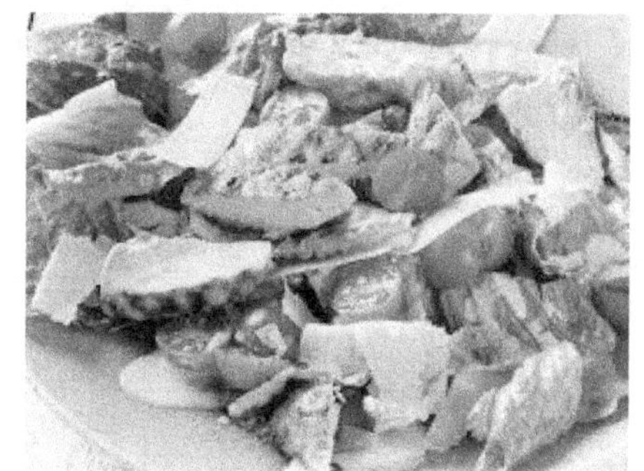

Preparation time : 5 minutes

Cooking time: 30 minutes

Servings: 4

Ingredients

1 cup sour cream

4-5 chicken breast halves

Salt to taste

Pepper to taste

1 cup feta cheese, crumbled

4 slices bacon

4 hard-boiled eggs, peeled, quartered

Serves: 4-5

Preparation

Place the chicken in a stockpot. Cover with cold water. Sprinkle salt.

Place the stockpot over medium heat. Cook until chicken is tender. Remove the chicken with a pair of tongs and place on your cutting board. Shred or chop into pieces.

Place a pan over medium heat. Add bacon and cook until brown.

Remove with a slotted spoon and place on a plate lined with paper towels. When cool enough to handle, chop into pieces.

Add chicken, bacon, and rest of the ingredients into a bowl and fold gently.

Chill and serve.

Nutrition: Calories: 189 Fat: 6.4g Carb: 3g Protein: 9.8g

Chapter 11: 21-day meal plan

DAY	BREAKFAST	LUNCH	DINNER
1.	Bacon-Wrapped Chicken Liver & Sage	Mongolian Beef Noodles	Turkey and Tomato Curry
2.	Bacon-Wrapped Garlic Chicken Bites	Slow Cooker Braised Beef	Stuffed Chicken Breast
3.	Bacon-Wrapped Salmon	Lamb Chops Pesto	Chicken Casserole
4.	Baked Bacon	Molasses and Mustard Flank Steak	Chicken-Stuffed Peppers
5.	Carnivore Breakfast Biscuits	Lime Coconut Skirt Steak	Crispy Chicken Thighs
6.	Carnivore Breakfast Pizza	Pork Chops Butternut Squash	BBQ Chicken Livers and Hearts
7.	Chicken Bacon Sausages	Slow Cooker Pot Roast	Lime Honey Chicken Skewers
8.	Cloud Cake Delight	Grilled Sweet Spicy Lamb Chops	Chicken with Cheesy Sauce
9.	Crispy Ham & Egg Cups	Steak Pineapple Rice	Buffalo Chicken Wraps
10.	Easy Egg & Bacon Cups	Rosemary Garlic Pork Chops	Taco Turkey Wraps
11.	Eggs & Bacon	Balsamic Orange Lamb Chops	Salt and Pepper Roast Chicken

12.	Eggs Poached in Stock	Pork Chops with Mushrooms	Parmesan Crusted Chicken Thighs with Bacon Cream Sauce
13.	Garlic Bacon-Wrapped Chicken Bites	Italian Pork Rolls	Simple, Pan-fried Chicken Breasts
14.	Hidden Treasure Meat Rounds	Thai Beef	Lemon Baked Salmon
15.	Keto Carnivore Waffle	Beef Pot Roast	Easy Blackened Shrimp
16.	Loaded Scrambled Eggs	Glazed Beef Meatloaf	The Best Garlic Cilantro Salmon
17.	Omelet with Bacon	Beef with Tzatziki	Aromatic Dover Sole Fillets
18.	Scotch Turkey Eggs	Meatballs with Mushroom Sauce	Trout with Butter Sauce
19.	Seared Bacon Burgers	Pan-Seared Duck Breast	Roasted Salmon
20.	Skillet Cooked Veal Cutlet for Brunch	Duck Breast with Vegetables	Salmon Meatballs
21.	Steak with Egg & Cheese	Duck Breast Salad	Grilled Oysters

Chapter 12: Meat protein and sport

The desire to kill is one of the main arguments. Carnivores love the smell of raw meat and the joy of catching live prey, killing it and consuming it wet. Human beings do not have this attribute and usually enjoy fruit and often eat apples, grapes or oranges just for their enjoyment and not because they are thirsty. This seems to suggest that fruit and vegetables are a natural diet for humans. We may eat meat, but we often don't kill it and eat it raw.

Some internal organs are also not used for the digestion of meat. Although all stomach secretions are acidic, carnivores have four times the acid content that humans do. This is what they need to break down their diet of flesh. These animals also have proportionately larger livers and kidneys to cope with an enormous amount of nitrogen contamination from a diet of meat. So, their liver secretes a lot of bile to cope with all the fat on the food. Carnivores are structurally appropriate for a normal diet of meat.

Most of us have a natural diet of fast food, including processed food and food containing preservatives, artificial flavor, color and very high sugar content. Some of the food we eat is so far away from the natural aspect that we don't even like the original; we just like the food that comes in a container or a bag. Such heavily processed products are typically very delicious, sometimes addictive and are always fattening. Also, food is full of artificial drugs, such as growth hormones and antibiotics, to protect pathogens from inhumane living conditions. Returning with nutrition back to its natural state would be a great help in maintaining good health and appropriate weight. Fresh vegetables, fruits, whole grains and non-fat yogurt or milk are nutritious foods that muscles and bones can use to make them stronger. We give good energy to exercise, which in effect, consumes fat.

Being and staying healthy relies on the nutrition we're consuming. If we need to lose weight, a well-balanced, low-calorie natural diet, with fresh fruits, vegetables and much of exercise, is the best way to do it. Extreme diets, synthetic fat burners, dietary supplements, and the most extreme of all, gastric bypass surgery are all ways to lose weight without really losing control of your life. You may remain a captive of the desire to eat food that is not at all helpful and possibly harmful to your wellbeing. Give a chance for freshness. It's going to change your life by making you safer, lighter, and hopefully, happy.

Benefits of body building

Bad health and anxiety are the kind of problems that affect everyone at some stage of their lives. They can be caused by many different reasons, but they can also be avoided, for the most part, by keeping our physical fitness in top shape. Exercise is well known for keeping your body fit, but it can also keep your mind in good condition. Brain, body and health benefits from physical fitness can be accomplished by daily outdoor exercise, as the sun can also work wonders for our wellbeing and mood.

Exercise can be beneficial as well as improving the flow of blood, increasing good feelings and helping to reduce negative feelings. Physical fitness advantages include surpassing the normal level of health, strengthening the immune system, promoting appetite to promote a lack of excess weight, and delivering an all-round sense of good health and vitality. Those who are physically fit often have more strength, are in better condition, and ultimately feel much happier and more comfortable than those who are lethargic and inactive.

One of the most important benefits to reaching the peak of physical fitness is the positive effect it has on the wellbeing of the body. Regular exercise can strengthen the heart, make it more effective and provide added protection against heart disease while lowering blood pressure, blood fats and bad cholesterol. There are many other advantages which come from reaching top physical fitness, but anything that enhances the body's most vital organ is probably the most significant achievement. Active activity through training helps in body strength and flexibility, bone strength and stress relief. The mental health effects of physical fitness are great, since exercise is well established to relieve stress and anxiety from the body, increasing a person's overall attitude and emotional state. It can help you sleep, and many symptoms can be changed when you work out such as PMS and tension headaches.

Only low levels of activity may benefit, particularly for those who are afraid to attend a gym or function in public. Activities such as gardening, walking, climbing stairs and even cleaning the house can be forms of exercise every day. Boring, regular exercises are not necessary to the attainment of physical fitness. Dancing and ice dancing are two fun ways to burn calories, boost muscle tone and step on to top physical activity. Even small changes can boost and lower the chances of disease or injury developing. These are few of the benefits that can be derived from reaching the peak of physical fitness.

They are over-nourished in Western society. We're hardly ever hungry. Our days are punctuated with meals, and most of us eat late at night, which is contrary to the way our bodies are designed to function. Animals will move faster and faster while their stomachs are clean, and in the days when we were hunters, this superior performance when we were starving added to our survival. Athletes will never exercise strenuously within a short time of taking food, and most of the exam candidates will tell you that they will get better results if they take an empty stomach exam. But we exist in an almost constant state of replenishment, a circumstance that was possibly incomprehensible to our predecessors, whose lives were dominated by sporadic starvation. The volume we consume and the kind of food we eat is most definitely linked to some of the killer diseases of our day.

There is a group living in northern Mexico where mortality from cardiovascular or circulatory failure is completely unknown. Such individuals are slim and tiny and weigh fewer than nine and a half stones on average. A daily calorie intake is well below the amount suggested by health authorities in developed countries who claim that Mexicans are undernourished. They will run races lasting forty-eight hours, while maintaining a steady speed of six miles an hour for more than 150 miles. They chase the deer until the animals fall out of exhaustion. Could it be that Western nutritionists are wrong and that these Mexicans are ideally nourished and we are over-nourished? There is no doubt at all that most of us eat a lot more than we need.

While almost every magazine we pick up has something to tell regarding food, calories and health, the basic truth is very plain. We need water, vitamins, minerals, proteins and calories to be healthy.

Calories: Three different kinds of food supply our calories: sugars, fats and proteins. Proteins and carbohydrates contain approximately the same amount of calories per ounce-about 100 as a rule of thumb. Fats, though, produce twice as much, so if you want to reduce your calorie intake, the obvious way to do this is to cut back on food. Fats, paradoxically, can sometimes help to regulate your hunger by sitting in your belly for a long time and giving you a feeling of replenishment.

What's a calorie, and why are diets and dieticians so focused on it? In caloric words, calorie is a measure of energy. So, a diet that contains a lot of calories per ounce offers you more fuel than one that has a small calorific value. In strict scientific terms, calorie is a calculation of heat and, in dietary terms, heat is fuel. Calories are essential in the diet, because if we do not eat all the calories we obtain in our food, the waste is stored as fat. The only way we can tell that we consume too many calories is by counting the number of calories we receive each day to lose weight. You need to take 3500 calories less than your body needs to lose a pound of weight. You lose it because your body burns its own fuel by taking its calories out of your fat.

If we eat food that contains more calories than we need, there's only one thing that can happen; we're going to gain weight. There is only one way to get rid of weight, and that is to consume fewer calories than we need. In doing so, we force our bodies to make up for the deficit by burning our own fat. We lose weight as we use our own fat. To maintain our weight stable, we need to consume the amount of food we require, in terms of calories, and not more.

The number of calories we use differs with gender (in fact, men need more than women because, on average, they are more active), with the job they do (manual work takes more calories than sedentary jobs), with age (we need more calories at twenty-five than at sixty), and with the manner we do it.

There is no doubt that some people consume calories more effectively than others. These are the lucky people who can consume whatever they like and stay thin. The less fortunate must be constantly careful about their diet. No one can change the rate at which their body metabolizes meat, and even though it appears that you're consuming very little, maybe significantly less than your mates, if you don't lose weight, you're actually eating more than you need, and you have to cut back even further. A lot of people who have a lean need and, of course, consume very little. Very often, they have a small appetite which serves as a buffer and decreases their usual intake of food to as little as a thousand calories a day without no effort whatsoever. Fat people, on the other side, usually have robust appetites that are not easily satisfied and more difficult to control. They seem to lack the 'I'm full' reflex.

Seek to include some of the following good examples as part of your own wellness campaign:

Get up early in the morning to get a jog

Walk or cycle to a shop or work rather than a car or a bus

Step up the stairs instead of using an elevator or a climber

Make other members of your family feel guilty when you exercise, and they don't

Meet your friends for a game of tennis or squash rather than a bar

Drink alcohol only at mealtimes (if you need to) and always in moderation

Encourage the friends not to consume too much liquor if they're driving home

Don't press other people with food or alcohol

Eat a lot of fish and vegetables

Don't eat two big meals a day. When dinner is set for the evening, consume just berries for breakfast or vice versa

Don't arrange your dinner party menu so that each course has high fat content

Provide salad and other healthy options as often as you can, particularly for slimmer's at dinner parties

Offer the friends and guests whole meal bread with' soft'-fat margarine instead of white bread and butter

Don't give sweets often to children of your own or other people

Don't offer as presents chocolates and candy and tobacco

If there are other citizens present, do not smoke without authorization

Compliment people for losing weight or giving up smoking

Don't sympathize or agree with people who say they can't stop smoking or lose weight

Don't praise a mom to a bony infant when the kid is small

Don't regard health as something that only doctors need to worry about

You'll feed on the carnivore diet until you're full. When you eat healthy, natural, satiating food, your body will not become a slave to sugar or an endless stream of unnecessary calories.

One helpful tip for us is to eat a sufficient amount of meat.

It's the answer for most people to eat more protein. But in the carnivore diet, too much protein can actually be harmful once you get enough.

If you have an insatiable hunger, you may not consume enough food. If this is you, then try eating fat for starvation, then apply protein to your muscles.

Most of the people end up consuming 1-2 pounds of meat a day.

Nevertheless, intermittent fasting is something to play with later on after a carnivorous diet. Moving from your current trash diet to both intermittent fasting and carnivorous diet would be pretty overwhelming, as both of them are big changes on their own.

It would much safer for them to get away with saying that carnivorous foods were unhealthy if people weren't:

– removing acne

– increasing strength

– repairing their intestines

– dropping 100+ pounds

– treating anxiety

– overcoming type 2 diabetes

Carnivore Diet Meal Plan & Shopping List

How to get going with that.

Now for some fun stuff. What does it feel like to feed a carnivore? Other than beautiful skin and infinite strength, of course.

This is an example of a week in the life of Carnivore Aurelius (cold showers and daily ultra-marathons have been written): to plan my shopping, I open an Excel spreadsheet and map out: how many meals I plan to eat of a certain food, and the amount of food per meal. Assuming that each meal consists of 16 oz of beef (you'll figure this out over time), I calculate the total amount to buy in buzz.

That, apparently, was just how our hunter-gatherer ancestors did it too...Based on the calendar above, you're going to have to buy the following sums in the right-hand column in the photo below.

If you're interested, here's a more comprehensive meal plan for carnivorous diets and a 30-day guide to getting started.

Using just animal products Servings: it extremely easy to run your weekly grocery shop. One of the basic selling points of the carnivore diet is how simple it is to obey.

Here is a list of foods licensed for carnivorous use: beef. The main source of calories will come from juicy cuts of grass-fed meat such as NY strip steak, porter, ribeye, 80/20 ground beef, T-bone, ham, pork chops and flank steak. Because you avoid carbs, meats with higher fat content are favored so that your body can use these fats as a useful source of energy.

Fish. Salmon, sardines, carp, mackerel and catfish are approved. Just like beef, target the fattest fish you can find.

Eggs, often regarded as multivitamin itself, are the ideal combination of meat, fat and essential body nutrients to keep your body working at its highest on a carnivorous diet.

Bone Marrow, bone broth is carnivorous-approved and is a great source of protein that also assists in the protection of the intestines, skin and joints.

Dairy, milk, grass-fed butter and cheese are technically allowed because they come from plants, but many carnivorous dieters try to keep milk intake to a minimal, as a large percentage of the population ultimately develops an allergy.

Conclusion

As you have reached the end of this book, first of all, I would like to thank you for using this guide to learn more about the carnivore diet. I hope you gained enough information to understand the advantages and disadvantages of following this diet alone. I am sure any meat lovers will definitely give it a go.

There are various online forums that you can find if you want to hear more from people who have already adopted the diet. You can also contact a physician to decide if the diet is appropriate for you; however, this diet is suitable and beneficial for you more often than not, especially in terms of weight loss. It may seem a bit tough to get through the first week or so of starting the diet, but you need to persevere through it.

The diet becomes very easy to follow after these initial days, and you're going to get used to it. Track your progress and calculate it both quantitatively and qualitatively when maintaining the diet.

We don't know enough about our safety. Eating healthy is a simple step you can take to improve your overall health.

Why you should eat healthier is to serve as fuel, you'll notice a huge difference in your energy levels and your balance during the day. Smarter food choices will give your body the strength you need to finish your daily tasks. If you've ever questioned why you're going to hit highs and lows in power all day, check at your diet and see if you're making smart food choices. Eating healthy can save you a lot of money, too!

It has been proven several times that a healthy food-fueled mind is more alert and can work at a higher level. I've seen the results of studies conducted on hundreds of average people, clear measures such as recall exercises and reaction cycles. We need to take care of ourselves to work at the highest level of performance. Making food choices healthier reduces your risk of diabetes, obesity, heart disease and some forms of cancer.

If you want to learn more from people who have already tried the diet, there are various online communities that you can find online. You can also consult your doctor while deciding if the diet is appropriate for you; however, more often than not, this diet is suitable and effective for you especially in terms of weight loss. The first week or so of starting the diet might seem a little tough to get through but you need to persevere through it.

After these initial days pass, the diet becomes very easy to follow and you will get used to it. While following the diet, track your progress and measure it quantitatively as well as qualitatively. Use this book as a guide while trying the carnivore diet and see how it works for you. If you find it useful, you can also go ahead and share or recommend it to family or friends who might benefit from following the carnivore diet too.

www.ingramcontent.com/pod-product-compliance
Lightning Source LLC
Chambersburg PA
CBHW081304250726
48662CB00008B/2393